THE FAT ELIMINATION AND DETOX PROGRAM (FED)

(A Holistic Approach to Disease Prevention and Weight Loss)

Jennifer A. Coscia, NC

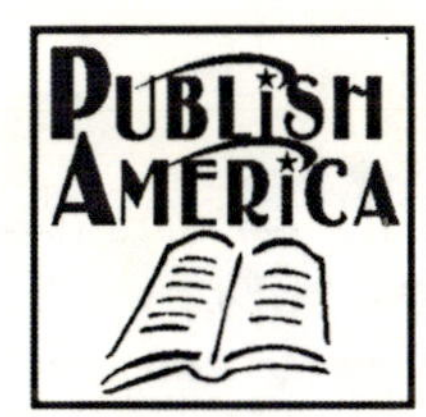

PublishAmerica
Baltimore

First printing

ISBN: 1-4137-5447-3
PUBLISHED BY PUBLISHAMERICA, LLLP
www.publishamerica.com
Baltimore

Printed in the United States of America

The information contained in this book has been derived from research, education, and observation of the author's clients and class participants, as well as personal experiences. It explains the correlation of certain food groups, diet supplements, and medications and how they affect our bodies. This book is solely to assist and guide you as you are educated on disease prevention strategies to attain optimal health and is by no means written to take the place of your personal physician or health-care professional. Consultation with your family physician is recommended before undergoing any exercise program, drastic changes to your diet or reduction in any medication. The author and publisher take no responsibility for any adverse effects that may arise from use or application of any information obtained in this book.

Table of Contents

Acknowledgments

I would like to offer my heartfelt appreciation to several people in my life that inspired me to write this book. First of all, I would like to thank my mother Mary Lou for all her help and dedication to this project. She is my greatest inspiration for writing this book. I would also like to acknowledge my dear friend Pam Samuels for her encouragement, support, and contribution to my work. Without her input I'm afraid this book would be just another resource guide for disease prevention and weight loss, instead of an autobiography of a lifetime of experience and education. I am also grateful to Clayton College of Natural Health, for the knowledge I attained pertaining to holistic medicine and nutrition. It truly opened my eyes to the many environmental problems of the world in which we live. And last, but certainly not least, I would like to thank my husband Michael, and daughter Arielle, for encouraging me to follow my dreams, and for being two of the greatest teachers in my life.

Jennifer A. Coscia, NC

Foreword

by C.W. Randolph, Jr., M.D.

I was honored when Jennifer Coscia first asked me if I would be willing to review this book in which she outlines a progressive and holistic approach to disease prevention and weight loss. I had long been impressed with Jennifer's comprehensive knowledge of how diet and nutrition can mingle with modern medicine and behavioral health to define a more integrated and personalized approach to healthcare. In addition, in my many discussions with Jennifer, I had found her explanations of the guiding principles behind her *Fat Elimination and Detox Program (FED)* to be clear and down to earth. Finally, as I read through the text, I was delighted with how Jennifer successfully blends her compassionate and informed voice with a unique perspective on health, disease, and their intimate relationship with each individual's responsibility. By the time I read the final chapter, I knew that this was a book that I would be privileged to both champion and recommend.

As a board-certified gynecologist, I have a very busy practice with a focus on women's health concerns and an emphasis on a more natural approach to medicine. I have a firsthand understanding of the critical roles that nutrition and nutritional biochemistry can play in disease prevention, as well as in defining one's overall health and well-being. Many times I have worked with patients who were astonished to learn that the underlying cause of a nagging health condition (often one that has defied previous attempts at diagnosis) could be linked back to their eating habits and inherent nutritional excesses or deficiencies. Like Jennifer, I have a strong belief that there is a real need to increase both the medical community's and the general public's awareness of the many benefits of holistic nutrition.

There is no arguing that our society eats too many empty calories and moves too little. According to a study released in 2003 by the United States Office of the Surgeon General, about three hundred thousand people die prematurely each year from being overweight. The number of obese American adults increased more than fifty percent between 1980 and 1994. In addition, obesity was identified as the second leading cause of death after smoking.

Why is weight gain such a problem? Why does the average American struggle to rein in their waistline? Jennifer's emphasis on a holistic approach to nutrition illuminates that "what we eat" is just part of the problem. Most people today do not perform physical labor to earn their wages. Instead, they are more sedentary, sitting at their desks in offices. This sedentary lifestyle is not conducive to increasing body metabolism and burning calories. Not having enough time in the day is also a contributing factor. More and more of my patients tell me that they rely on fast foods and pre-packaged, processed meals, because they don't have the time or energy to go to the grocery store, purchase fresh ingredients, and prepare a meal at the end of a busy day.

The medical community is well aware of how obesity is linked to many chronic diseases. We know that being overweight increases a person's risk for a number of serious ailments, including diabetes, heart disease, strokes, high blood pressure, and some types of cancer. What we don't know is how to address the problem. Advising someone to lose weight sounds simple. However, as Jennifer so appropriately points out throughout this book, taking that advice is easier said than done. Even more tragic is the fact that many well-intentioned individuals bounce between the latest "fad" diets and starve themselves. Chronic dieters actually do their bodies harm by denying themselves the essential nutrients that should be part of a healthy diet. As I read this book's first chapter and saw the words, "You must EAT FOOD to lose weight," I wanted to stop and give Jennifer a standing ovation. The reality is that humans must eat to obtain the necessary fuel to thrive. The question that most of us struggle with, however, is what should we eat and how much? The question of "what to eat" is much more complex than it may appear at first glance and requires a more in-depth examination of our dietary choices. Today, fat-laden animal products (lacking in fiber and nutrients) are more commonly seen at our meals than fresh fiber-rich, plant-based foods. Moreover, our fast-moving culture has fostered many new businesses revolving around non-nutritious and highly-processed ingredients. While the high level of consumer demand for quick meals and snacks has made food refinement a successful industry, it has also fostered a new way of eating that has many deleterious health effects.

As Jennifer aptly points out, the average American is bombarded with chemicals and toxins that are ever present in our air, water, and the food we eat. Medical research has proven that over time these toxins can depress the body's immune system, reduce fertility rates, and even serve as a precursor for cancer. The readers of this book will be provided with fundamental knowledge of how the foods they consume will impact their health. Jennifer then goes on to give practical advice on how to eat nutritionally and how to eliminate toxins from the body. She offers guidance on food choices and gives the reader parameters for determining food quantities.

As a physician, I am gratified that Jennifer spells out for the reader the exact reasons that she feels it is wise (and often necessary) to improve our diet. A nutritionally sound diet, along with nutritional supplementation, is vital for maintaining our health under the onslaught of stress (both physical and environmental), the many toxins in our lives, and the advancement of age. Her specific dietary recommendations make this book a "how-to" guide for anyone seeking to improve their health while losing weight. In an era where most of our healthcare systems are still vested in treating sick people, Jennifer's emphasis on preventative health and individual choice is refreshing.

Finally, Jennifer outlines her FED program in a way that acknowledges that we are all human. She empathized with the fact that the average person has a life that requires the multi-tasking of daily activities rather than a life lending to the rhythm of simplicity. I felt comforted when I read her words:

"At any given time, we should do the best we can at that time. Some times are going to be easier and better than others, and that's okay."

In closing, I want to congratulate Jennifer on her efforts to return our focus to one of the most primary and essential contributors to our health: what we choose to eat. Jennifer Coscia's FED Program has the potential to re-shape a perception of the term diet from one of loss to a term that connotes better health. I hope that as others read this book they will also recognize the wisdom of her holistic approach to nutrition and disease prevention.

Introduction

Reflection

For as long as I can remember, there have been "fad"diets. I have tried most of them and unfortunately, most of them failed. They would work for a short time, but soon the weight would find its way back to me. I managed to find one that worked fairly well and I slowly lost sixty pounds. I have successfully kept the weight off, staying within fifteen pounds of my goal weight, for over fifteen years. Because I liked the program so much, I became an instructor for this weight loss organization. I soon realized that this diet did not work well for everyone and it frustrated me that my weight- loss members would tell me how well they adhered to the plan, yet they would continue to gain weight and really struggled to lose it. Years later, having attained a degree in holistic nutrition, I finally understood why diets would work for some and not for others. Everyone is different. We are all ninety-nine point nine percent physiologically the same. However, that point one percent is what makes us individual. There is no one "fix" for everyone, especially when it comes to dieting. As a result of my education and experiences, I realized how unhealthy these weight-loss programs could be. Artificial sweeteners, low-fat foods with additives, processed foods, and high-sodium frozen meals eventually took their toll on my body. It has taken a long time to undo the damage I did from unhealthy weight-loss programs.

There are plenty of diet plans on the market today. There are some that work really well, until you start eating certain foods again. Others tax the liver because of protein overload, causing the depletion of vital nutrients. The fact is, we have to go back to basics to lose weight; and the simplicity of it will astound you.

I have also found that to be truly successful at weight loss, you must first learn to be realistic about your target goal weight. Weight is only a number. How you feel at a certain healthy weight is what matters most, not what a chart shows you should weigh. The mind must also get over the sensationalism of fad diets, and the unrealistic portrayal of how we are supposed to look. The unrealistic expectations of wanting to look "model thin" or "muscle bound" can lead to frustration and eventually failure. There are many factors to take into consideration before choosing your goal weight, such as gender, age, and frame size. *The Fat Elimination and Detox Program (FED)* is based on the individual's basal metabolic rate (BMR). Later on, I'll explain how to calculate your BMR (basal metabolic rate) and your BMI (body mass index). These numbers are very important to the success of your weight loss, as you will discover later on in the book.

Learning to eat the proper foods, along with taking synergistic supplements, to encourage weight loss, is what the FED program is all about. In addition, taking the FED program one day at a time, one pound at a time, is a key component to the success of your disease preventative weight-loss journey.

Obesity and Toxins in a Chemical World

Dr. Tazewell Banks, the director of the Heart Program at DC General, once said it would be better if parents told their children to go out and play in traffic than allow children to eat foods rich in saturated fats found in fast-food restaurants. Saturated and hydrogenated fats are the culprits when it comes to high cholesterol and vascular congestive problems. The number one disease related to the increase in dietary fat is arteriosclerosis, better known as the clogging of the coronary arteries. Arteriosclerosis causes the most deaths in Western "diet" cultures. Chronic diseases, such as heart disease and many cancers are now at an all-time high, affecting millions of people of all ages. I remember (as a young girl growing up in the '70s) how scarce the word cancer was in our household. Cancer and heart disease were diseases for the aged, certainly not for young people. Unfortunately today, during my seminars on disease prevention, when I ask the question, "How many of you have cancer or heart disease in your immediate or extended family?" at least eighty percent of those attending the class raise their hands. I then ask them to leave their hands up and to the rest of the group ask, "How many of you know someone with either cancer or heart disease?" This time, sadly to say, I have full participation of the class. There is something greatly wrong with those statistics.

Today, the world in which we live is far from perfect, thanks to industry.

Industrial disasters, such as Love Canal and Times Beach, Missouri, in which the environmental negligence of chemical manufacturing plants took place, caused the suffering of many. The news of these devastating "accidents" soon spread across the nation and we were rudely awakened to the environmental dangers of modernized industry and the multitude of problems they created. These dangers were not visible or even known to most of us. Nonetheless, they were ever present in our environment and unfortunately remain there even today.

According to J. Robert Hatherhill, Ph.D., author of *Eat to Beat Cancer*, there are over one hundred thousand chemicals used in industry today. We have over six hundred chemicals in our bodies that were not present prior to 1900 and over one thousand more than our ancestors did over five hundred years ago. One new chemical enters industrial use every twenty minutes. Pesticides and herbicides continue to wreak havoc on our environment. In 1976 there were over forty thousand pesticide products available. That number has nearly doubled today. Even with the elimination of DDT in 1973, it is still turning up in far regions of the world in soil testing. That means that the very food we grow can still be contaminated even without the use of harmful chemicals. Our environment, homes, schools, churches, and businesses are full of carcinogens (cancer-causing agents) and toxic chemicals. Unfortunately, most of us are completely unaware of the many health problems they cause. Dry cleaning solvents, household cleaning agents, paints and varnishes, cosmetics, food additives, carpeting, pharmaceutical drugs, and animal products, such as meat and dairy, are just a few of the many toxins in our lives.

Do these toxins make us fat? Many of these chemicals are fat soluble, which means they need fat to be dissolved, so these chemicals store in tissue that is high in fat. Synthetic chemicals used to fatten livestock for meat production by reducing their ability to use their own fat stores, does indeed contribute to weight gain in humans from the consumption of their meat. Animals fed organophosphates (growth promoters) gain weight while consuming less food. We, in turn, ingest these growth promoters and antibiotics from eating meat. Even though use of growth promoters has been banned in parts of Europe, when researchers found them to be highly toxic, the United States refused to heed the warning. Organophosphates remain in use by means of pesticides, gasoline additives, rubber, and lubricating oil. Once these organophosphates get into your system, they will continue to make it harder for you to lose weight and possibly make you gain weight, even though you are consuming less food. One of the many reasons why this happens is because the liver cannot efficiently metabolize fat if it is overloaded with toxins and pollutants.

Something has to be done in this war against cancer, and other chronic diseases, and it has to begin with you. You and you alone have the power to change the way you and your family live by reducing known carcinogens and toxins in your lives, beginning with the food you eat. This is probably the most important change to adapt into your life. After all, you are literally what you eat!

The Fat Elimination and Detox Program (FED) was designed as a disease prevention program. FED will also help you chose an ideal weight and achieve that goal safely and effectively without pills or starvation. The many foods you will be eating are specific foods for disease prevention that are geared at burning fat while fueling the body. Some of these foods will act as medicine in the body, helping to ward off disease by lowering cholesterol and high blood pressure and will even help to balance blood sugar levels. Adults and children will greatly benefit from the FED program. To ensure a healthy outcome, this program involves some lifestyle changes and a whole new way of eating. The whole body connection will thrive and your life will never be the same. Change is one of the hardest things we must endure, but it is a vital necessity in life. Eat well, live well, and be well!

Chapter One

The Holistic Approach, Why We Need It

Holistic simply means the "whole" body. If you were to look up the word holistic, in the dictionary, it would say it is a philosophy based on the principle that everything in nature, such as complete individuals and other complete organisms function as a complete unit that cannot be reduced to the sum of their parts. The lack of incorporating this principle is one of the many problems with modern (Western) medicine today. In general physicians don't bother to look at the whole picture. Instead their approach to medicine is to only look at symptoms that are apparent at the time of the patient's office visit. What are medical records for if no one bothers to look at them? There is valuable information in one's medical records such as, previous illnesses and injuries, family history, and most importantly, medications. Without this prior knowledge how can a physician possibly know the whole needs of the patient? A person could be sent from specialist to specialist, and oftentimes endure unnecessary testing with each physician not knowing what the other one is doing. Medications are at times carelessly prescribed without knowing current or previous medications, which in turn can be hazardous to the patient. Many of these patients have numerous contraindications with diet, supplements, and other medications. I know too many people who have been caught up in this vicious cycle. It is easy to get lost in the shuffle and frustrated with the process. I will elaborate more on contraindications for medications, herbs, and supplements later in the book.

I remember awhile back, I went to see a gastroenterologist for a pain in my stomach that was quite bothersome. I knew he would want to put me through a barrage of tests, so I thought ahead and brought copies of the tests my primary care doctor had already ordered. When I started to show him the test results, beginning with a full blood panel, he abruptly retorted, "I am not a hematologist.

I explained to him that I thought he might want to get the "whole picture" by taking a look at my other test results. He just ignored me. I thought that he might have noticed something amiss in my results that could possibly have saved me from undergoing unnecessary tests. Needless to say, seeing that physician was a waste of time. Later that week, I went to see a recommended acupuncture practitioner, who treated me with a holistic approach. Three weeks and three visits later the pain was gone. I had an infection that involved the pyloric sphincter valve, located between my stomach and duodenum, which may explain the reason why my white cell count was slightly elevated in my blood panel report. What she did that was so out of the ordinary for the Western medicine approach, was she listened to everything I had to say about myself pertaining to my problem, including past medical history. She then charted and tested my whole body for weaknesses. I was thrilled that I didn't have to go through an upper GI series, ultrasound, and an endoscopy, which was what the gastroenterologist prescribed, along with medications. I was leery about taking medications before diagnosis and was rapidly growing tired of the "Band-Aid syndrome mentality" that was vastly becoming popular with Western medicine. This simply is the process of prescribing medications for symptoms instead of getting to the root of the problem. All this achieves is to cover up the initial problem and in turn creates other problems from the adverse reactions of the prescribed medication. That pretty much sums up a visit to the doctor's office nowadays. I read that there are over one hundred and fifty prescriptions written for every one hundred patients seen. Western medicine certainly has its place. However I feel there is definitely room for improvement. A holistic approach to medicine would be a great place to start.

Nutritional Basics

By looking at the whole picture with a holistic view, we can begin to delve into all aspects of the body, beginning with a basic grasp on nutrition.

The word nutrition is used twofold. Here is a little Biology 101 to help you understand the complexity of the human body when it comes to nutrition.

First, nutrition is considered a science that seeks to comprehend food, its nutrients, how nutrients are used by the body, and how improper amounts or combinations can lead to illness. Nutrition is also the term that describes all the processes in which we take food in and utilize it, including ingestion, digestion, absorption and assimilation. Ingestion simple means consuming food. The actual process of eating, including chewing, is the beginning of digestion. The average person only chews each bite eleven to twenty-six times before swallowing, when in actuality you should chew each bite sixty to one hundred times. When you chew your food efficiently you release natural enzymes within the food that will aid digestion. When consuming a meal you should always sit down and take the time to enjoy your food. Eating a meal on the run can result in all sorts of digestive upsets, the foremost being, indigestion. It also causes us to overeat, because the brain doesn't have enough time to register that we've had enough. You are better off not eating at all during a stressful or hectic moment. Put your meal off until you can take time to eat slowly and calmly to ensure proper digestion. Digestion is the breakdown of complex food molecules to simpler molecules. Some people are under the misconception that hydrochloric acid digests food. Hydrochloric acid creates an acidic environment so that enzymes such as, pepsin, which breaks down protein, can thrive and do their job. Hydrochloric acid does, however, aid the breakdown of certain chemicals. Absorption is the movement of simple molecules from the digestive system to the circulatory system for disbursement throughout the body. Assimilation, on the other hand, involves the transformation and incorporation of molecules into the structure of the organism.

Macronutrients

Macronutrients are referred to as the "big" picture in nutrition. Macronutrients include proteins, fats, carbohydrates, fiber and water.

Protein is an essential element in nutrition. It makes up about twenty percent of our body weight and is the key component for muscles, nails, hair, skin, eyes and internal organs. Our blood (hemoglobin) and hormones are protein, as well as, our immune defense system. Growth and the maintenance of body tissue also requires protein, especially during childhood, pregnancy and lactation. However, as I mentioned before, we can overdose on too much protein. There is a simple method to determine what your personal protein ratio should be for your body weight. Take your body weight and multiply it by .45. A person that weighs 160 pounds should consume approximately 72 grams of protein daily. To give you an idea of how overzealous we Americans are with our protein intake, here is an average American daily account of protein. Having a three-egg omelet with ham and cheese for breakfast, an American sub for lunch made with cheese, ham, turkey and roast beef, and a barbecue chicken dinner, contains over 140 grams of protein! That's double the recommended protein intake. Unlike carbohydrates and fats, protein cannot be stored. As I mentioned before, too much protein intake taxes the liver to the point where it can no longer metabolize fat or aid in the removal of pollutants and environmental toxins. This wreaks havoc on our entire system. Be wary of diets that promote high-protein and low-carbohydrate foods. There is, however, a flip side to this coin. Many people, over the age sixty, don't consume an adequate amount of protein. This can lead to a disorder called sarcopenia, which means flesh loss. Sarcopenia usually begins around the age of forty-five when muscle mass starts to decrease. This is caused by the decrease of hormones that promote muscle growth, which coincides with the fact that physical activity also declines at this age, creating additional muscle loss and weakness. It is strongly advised for people over fifty-five to consume at least .45 grams of protein per pound of body weight. Protein food sources would include meats, poultry, fish, eggs, milk, cheese, nuts, seeds, and legumes.

Carbohydrates are probably the most important of the macronutrients since they are our main source of energy and should constitute fifty percent of the diet. As I mentioned before, the major shift that began in the 1950s with the widespread refinement of food, leads us away from the healthful consumption of fresh fruits and vegetables and complex carbohydrates and toward a diet of more refined carbohydrates and simple sugars. I will elaborate on this later in the book. This shift is responsible for a number of diseases, among them obesity, diabetes, cardiovascular disease, and many types of cancers. Carbohydrates are a quick source of energy for the body because they are easily converted into glucose, which is the fuel for the body's many cells. Each gram of carbohydrate releases four calories, which are units of heat or energy. Carbohydrates not only fuel the body but they are also responsible for the regulation of fat and protein metabolism. Along with protein and fat, carbohydrates help the immune system fight infections, promote growth of body tissues, including bones and skin, and lubricate joints. Many carbohydrate foods are also high in fiber, which is instrumental in the prevention of many diseases, especially those related to the colon, such as colon cancer, hemorrhoids, constipation, diverticulosis and obesity.

Fiber, also helps lower blood cholesterol levels, stabilize blood sugar levels, and aids in the removal of toxic metals from the body. The recommended daily amount of fiber is at least twenty-five grams. To ensure you meet this requirement, consume plenty of these high-fiber foods, whole grains including oat, wheat, corn, rye, and rice, and flours, brown rice, bran, most fresh fruit, dried fruit, nuts, seeds (flaxseeds are beneficial), beans, lentils, peas, and fresh vegetables. Once again, I must reiterate that carbohydrates are a vital part of the diet and are essential for life.

Fat, is probably the "star" of macronutrients. It is certainly the most talked about and deliberated over. Do we need fat in our diet? Assuming the answer is yes, then how much? What kinds are best? What happens when they're heated? All of these questions seem to constantly come up and depending on whom you ask, the answers will vary. The fact of the matter is we definitely need fat in our diet. We should consume, at the very least, twenty percent of our calories from good healthy fats. Where most weight loss plans are deficient in this macronutrient, the American diet is in excess. In children, fat is needed for normal brain development and throughout life it is needed to supply energy and support growth. Fat is actually the most concentrated source of energy available to our body. A gram of fat is nine calories, whereas, protein and carbohydrates are only four calories per gram. After two years of age, the body only requires a small amount of fat, and once again, the American diet supersedes these requirements. Excess fat intake is implicated in many diseases such as, obesity, coronary heart disease, certain cancers, and high blood pressure.

To understand the reasoning behind fats and disease, you must first understand the different types of fat and the way they act within the body. Let's begin with saturated fats. Saturated fatty acids are usually found in animal products, such as dairy products and meat. The fat you see in meat is saturated. Palm kernel oil, coconut oil, and vegetable shortening are also saturated fats. The liver uses saturated fats to manufacture cholesterol; therefore excessive dietary intake of saturated fat can significantly raise blood cholesterol levels, especially the bad cholesterol, LDL, low-density lipoproteins. Polyunsaturated fatty acids are found in flax, corn, soybean, safflower, sunflower, and in certain fish oils. They can actually help to lower cholesterol levels, although, large amounts tend to reduce good cholesterol HDLs, as well. Monounsaturated fatty acids are found in vegetable and nut oils, such as olive, peanut and canola oils. They seem to lower LDL levels, without affecting the good cholesterol HDLs. Another much talked about topic is trans-fatty acids, they are responsible for raising LDL (bad) cholesterol levels, also known as trans fats, these substances occur when polyunsaturated oils are altered through the process of hydrogenation, a process used to harden liquid vegetable oils into solid foods like margarine and shortening. Flaxseed (polyunsaturated), olive and canola oil (monounsaturated) are the best choices, however, flaxseed oil is not appropriate for cooking as it is easily damaged by heat. I'll discuss more on the importance of fat later on.

Water, the final macronutrient we will discuss, is something we need on a regular basis to sustain life. We can go weeks without food, however, water is a different story. You would die within a couple of days without water. Our body is approximately sixty-five percent water. All chemical reactions, in living things, take place in water and water is the primary source of our lymph, blood, and body tissue fluids. Did you know that when you are thirsty that you're already in the early stages of dehydration? This is why it is important to drink six to eight glasses of good clean water daily. Good, clean water is hard to come by these days. Make sure your water source is pure. Contaminated water is a known carcinogen and disease promoter for diseases such as, cancers of the bladder and rectum (over fifteen thousand cases annually), and infectious disease like, E.coli and cryptosporidium. Tap water is the biggest offender. Today your tap water may be contaminated with bacteria, viruses, trihalomethanes (THMs), and other pathogens. This also includes beverages made from municipal water from orange juice to beer. THMs occur from water that has been contaminated with organic compounds prior to chlorination, which turns these organic compounds into carcinogens. Bottled water is also known to be contaminated. To be sure your favorite spring water isn't contaminated do some homework. Contact the supplier and request monitoring reports, or better yet, perform your own test at home. You can buy a water-testing kit from your local hardware store, and while you are at it, purchase a good filter for your kitchen faucet and for your shower head to safeguard yourself against THMS, bacteria, viruses, arsenic, lead, fluoride, chlorine, aluminum, pesticides, industrial pollutants, and radioactive contaminants. Your skin is your second lung so bathing in contaminated water can still harm you. You can also contact your local water testing company to have your water tested. From a health perspective, I can't stress enough the importance of clean water. I am a firm believer that our drinking water is one of the many contributing factors of chronic disease.

Basal Metabolic Rate

Foods and beverages we consume on a daily basis are what constitute a person's diet. A diet must contain a sufficient amount of all macronutrients to maintain the body and sustain life. If one's diet is deficient in nutrients, or if for some reason a person cannot process nutrients efficiently, a dietary deficiency and illness will result. Large amounts of energy are required for muscular activity, however, even at rest energy is required for breathing, heart rate, and other normal body functions. Your basal metabolic rate, (BMR), is the rate at which the body uses energy when at rest. There are several factors that affect a person's BMR. Basal metabolic rates decline throughout life, with children having the highest rate and the elderly having the lowest. Generally speaking, men have a higher BMR than most women. Height and weight are also important factors. Many adults will fall into the range of 1200-2200 calories for their basal metabolic rate. It is very important to know what yours is. This will tell you the minimum amount of calories you personally should consume to sustain life. Many people, including myself, thought that less is more when dieting. If we eat less, then technically, we should lose weight. Right? Wrong! If you consume fewer calories than your basal metabolic rate, your body will think you're trying to starve it, so the body will become very greedy with incoming calories and will hold onto them. A while ago I decided to go on a quick diet to lose eight to ten pounds. I thought to myself, no problem. I ate all the right foods, exercised religiously, drank my water and nothing happened, no weight loss and I swear I even gained a pound or two! How could this be? Well, I decided to find out what my BMR was. I was shocked when I learned that I needed to consume at least 1400 calories daily. I was consuming only about 1000 calories a day and did I mention that I was exercising like an exercise addict? I was easily burning 500 calories a day. So let's do the math. I was taking in 1000 calories and burning or using up 500 calories. That means that I was only giving my body 500 calories to sustain existence. I essentially went into what is called survival mode, which will eventually take its toll on your body. You must EAT FOOD to lose weight. To find out your BMR, the following equation is known as the Harris-Benedict Equation. (It isn't as difficult as it looks. If you have a problem, you can get an average BMR by multiplying your weight by ten. Example: 145 x 10 = 1450 BMR.) Keep in mind though, the equation has three variables to factor in such as, weight, height, and age.

Women: (BMR)

Divide your weight by 2.2,
then multiply sum by 9.6 = sum
Multiply your height in inches by 2.54,
then multiply sum by 1.7 = sum
Multiply your age by 4.7 = sum
+ 655
sum of weight + sum of height - sum of age + 655 = BMR
(Make sure you subtracted your age NOT added it.)

Example: 145 divided by 2.2 = 64.9
Multiplied by 9.6 = 623.0
66 inches multiplied by 2.54 = 167.6 Multiplied by 1.7 = 284.9
40 years multiplied by 4.7 = 188
+ 655

623.0 + 284.9 - 188 + 655 = 1375 BMR

Men: (BMR)

Divide your weight by 2.2,
then multiply sum by 13.7 = sum
Multiply your height in inches by 2.54,
then multiply by 5 = sum
Multiply your age by 6.8 = sum
+ 66
sum of weight + sum of height - sum of age + 66 = BMR
(Make sure you subtracted your age NOT added it.)

Example: 180 divided by 2.2 = 81.8
multiplied by 13.7 = 1120.6
72 multiplied by 2.54 = 182.8
multiplied by 5 = 914.4
45 years multiplied by 6.8 = 306
+66
1120.6 + 914.4 - 306 + 66 = 1795 BMR

As previously mentioned, over sixty percent of Americans are overweight or obese. Why is weight control such a major problem for such a large portion of our population? There are several metabolic pathways that convert carbohydrates (glucose) or proteins to fat. Stored body fat was very important to our prehistoric ancestors because it helped them survive long periods when food was scarce. During these times of food scarcity, stored fat could be used to supply energy. Today, however, food scarcity is not a problem for most of us; and even small amounts of excess food, eaten daily, can ADD to our fat stores. Energy doesn't weigh anything, but the nutrients that contain energy do. *Weight control is the art of balancing the calories we take in and the energy we burn through normal daily routines and exercise;* and that, pretty much sums it up. There is a limit to the rate at which a person can use body fat as an energy source. On average, a person can lose one to three pounds of body fat a week when dieting, safely. One pound of fatty tissue contains approximately 3500 calories. If you have a BMR of 1600 calories daily, you must take into consideration that any exercise you do must be accounted for, by adding those calories burned back into the equation. Here we go again with math (not my favorite subject). If you have a BMR of 1600 calories daily, and you are exercising causing your body to use up 300 calories, then you must add those burned calories back into your caloric intake making that total number 1900. This way your body doesn't think you are trying to starve it. This is very important if you plan to be successful with your weight-loss program. Safe consistent weight loss should be one to three pounds per week. Keep in mind that your BMR (basal metabolic rate) is the minimum amount of calories that you should consume daily. So, rule of thumb would be to use your actual BMR as your starting point for weight loss. It's really very simple once you understand it. The FED Program is designed specifically for balancing caloric intake and usage.

Body Mass Index

A useful guideline to determine if you are overweight is by determining your body mass index (BMI), your appropriate body weight compared to your height. This is very easy to figure out. Take your weight and multiply it by 703, then take that sum and divide it by your height in inches, twice. For example, a woman that weighs 170 pounds and is five- foot six- inches would have a BMI of 27.4 (170 pounds multiplied by 703 equals 119510, divided by sixty-six inches equals 1810.75, divided by sixty-six again equals 27.4). What this means is that this woman is considered overweight. A healthy normal range should be between 18.5 and 24.9. Those with a BMI between 25 and 29.9 are considered overweight and those with a BMI of 30 or more are obese.

Fad Diets with Short-term Results

There are numerous diets that promise large and rapid weight loss but unfortunately, only result in temporary weight/water loss. This is due to the fact that some diet plans encourage eating and drinking foods that are diuretics, which in turn increases the amount of urine produced to promote water loss. Low carbohydrate, high-protein diets deprive the body of glucose, which is needed for nerves, tissue, and red blood cells among many other things. When this happens the body begins to use protein from the liver and muscles in order to provide sufficient glucose for these vital cells. This type of weight loss is not healthy for anyone, and weight loss from a temporary fast (a form of starvation), results from the stomach and digestive tract, being empty. I personally have dropped five pounds on a two-day fast, however, as soon as I started eating food again my weight came right back up. I am a promoter of fasting for certain health reasons, primarily because it helps to rid the body of toxins. Be aware of so-called quick weight-loss diet plans. Find out how the diet will affect your body in the long run. Is this plan something you can continue for life without jeopardizing your health? Yo-yo dieting is dangerous for your health, whereas maintaining a healthy weight is beneficial. Subtle fluctuations in weight are expected. This holds true especially for women, which is due to their menstrual cycles. It is not uncommon to fluctuate three to five pounds a month due to water weight gain. There are many diets on the market today that are very unrealistic, not something you could sink your teeth into and get excited about. Some become too regimented or monotonous and eventually we get bored, tired, frustrated and end up quitting or surrendering back to our old habits. A good, healthful diet program should be something you can attain and adjust accordingly, for life.

Testimonial

BEVERLY

My name is Beverly and over the years I slowly gained weight. Every year a few more pounds were added and before I knew it I was overweight. In January of 2001, I had to have two stents put in my heart; I had high blood pressure, high cholesterol, and had no energy. I was also on several medications. I knew it was time for me to take control of my body. I had heard about the FED program and invited Jennifer Coscia to bring her program to my place of business. She encouraged me and gave me support. I lost over fifteen pounds in eight weeks. In addition, my blood pressure and cholesterol levels dropped significantly, I regained my energy, and I am working on decreasing my medications. This life changing experience is just the beginning for me. I will continue using the FED program as a new way of life and will encourage others to do the same. Thank you, Jennifer!

Chapter Two

Chronic Disease, Out Of Control

A hundred years ago our ancestors consumed a simple diet that consisted of fresh fruits, vegetables and grains. Meat and most other animal products were hard to come by and oftentimes, expensive. Farming was very different from the farming industry of today. Harsh carcinogenic pesticides and herbicides didn't exist. Life was hard, but a lot less complicated than present times. Heart disease and cancers were a rarity, so rare that medical textbooks failed to mention them up through the late 1800s. Today, heart disease is the number one killer. In the year 2000 cardiovascular disease (CVD) was responsible for one out of every two point five deaths in the United States. That amounts to over one million deaths annually. Cancer claimed the lives of over five hundred and fifty thousand Americans that same year. What happened to those less complicated times when cancer and heart disease barely existed? Something went drastically wrong between the late 1800s and today. As we look back through history at the evolution of "the Western diet," you will see exactly where we went wrong.

Industry

Progress began with the replacement of farming horses for the modern convenience of tractors. Horses could prepare several acres for planting in one day, whereas, tractors could plow fifty acres a day. There was no contest and plow horses were soon "put out to pasture" (so to speak), except for those few farmers that fought progress and stayed with traditional means. America was rapidly becoming a mechanized industrial country, employing petroleum-based fertilizers and pesticides to extend crop yields. We soon replaced a traditional diet with animal products loaded with fat and lacking fiber and vital nutrients, which took the place of fresh fiber-rich plant-based foods. Animal products began to dominate the majority of our meals.

Shortly thereafter, we introduced the refinement of food with the use of roller mills to process grains, followed by the canning industry (that was blanching food with heat), again destroying vital nutrients prior to sealing it up in metal tins. Certain foods can absorb up to eighty percent of the metals from the cans they are contained in. During the mid 1900s, widespread refinements to food became our main focus, bringing food-processing factories across America. As television became the American staple, food manufacturers responded with highly processed, non-nutritious, frozen TV dinners. Television, radio, and magazine ads were everywhere, tantalizing us at every turn. I remember as a kid what a treat it was to be able to sit down in front of the television, with a TV dinner, and watch our favorite program.

To limit bacteria that would cause spoilage, foods were heated to high temperatures in processing. The heating process killed the bacteria, but it also destroyed natural anti-cancer agents, forming carcinogenic chemicals in the process. To top that off, in order to add taste and texture to food, the industry began experimenting with literally thousands of additives. The industrial revolution began introducing artificial chemicals for the first time in our planet's history. By the mid '80s, the National Research Council estimated that there were over five million chemical compounds made by various chemical industries. Today, as I stated earlier, it is possible to detect over six hundred different chemicals in our bodies that were not present prior to 1900.

Toxic America

We have finally realized the impact of toxicity caused by the many chemicals in use today; yet we are still continually exposed to them in our food, air, and water. It is not by our choice, and unfortunately everyone on the planet is exposed to these toxins. How do these toxins affect us? In the early 1950s, we began to change the way livestock were grown in the United States. Chickens were fed nutrient-rich and additive-laden, antibiotic-culture waste called growth promoters or growth hormones (as we know them today), to make them fatter faster; and chicken growers reaped the harvest getting more money for less output. Growth promoters have now become a multimillion-dollar business. Several countries in Europe have already banned the use of growth promoters because of the many health threats associated with their use. Over half of the antibiotics manufactured in the

United States today go directly to the feed of poultry, pigs, and beef cattle. As a result, feeding antibiotics to livestock is causing antibiotic-resistant bacteria to develop and spread; and the massive overuse of antibiotics on livestock is directly responsible for the increase in human infectious diseases. We in turn, consume these chickens and other livestock, thus ingesting these dangerous antibiotic-resistant bacteria.

Technology had also led to rapid changes in the diet of many countries in the developed world. With the evolution of agricultural technology at hand, we were able to produce and store many different foods. There has never before, in history, been such a wide variety of crops available to us, yet most of the industrialized diet is packaged and loaded with fat (especially hydrogenated oils) and sugar. The actual packaging of food also poses health risks because of possible contaminants, toxins and poisons. Canned goods and food wraps, in particular, may contain lead. Lead has recently been associated with learning disabilities, such as Attention Deficit Disorder (ADD), and aggressive behavior. Lead also shows up in paint, paint dust, colored newsprint, soil and water. Rice and vegetables cooked in lead-contaminated water will absorb eighty percent of the lead.

While on the subject of hazardous metals, I'd like to make you aware of the many metals that can affect our bodies. Cadmium is found in our diet by means of organ meats like liver and kidney, and has been linked to Parkinson's disease. Shellfish like snails, shrimp, oysters, mussels, crab and some fish, tend to have high amounts of cadmium from being exposed, while in their environment on the ocean floor. Cadmium is a metal that accumulates in soft tissues, especially the kidneys, and has been linked to many chronic diseases, including kidney disease and prostate cancer. Cigarettes are another source of cadmium; and smoking a pack a day can double the amount of absorbed cadmium in the body. Mercury, another metal that is found in fish and seafood, is easily absorbed through diet, again due to the mercury levels in water. Any fish with teeth that feeds on other fish will have higher levels of mercury and polychlorinated biphenyls (PCBs). PCBs cause many health problems because its' primary target is the immune system. A study last year in the *New England Journal of Medicine* linked heart disease in men with increased mercury levels from consuming contaminated fish. Heart attack sufferers had fifteen percent higher levels of mercury than those with no history of heart disease.

Therefore, you should try to consume deepwater fish like halibut, flounder, tuna, cod, and salmon. Albacore tuna is extremely high in mercury, so be sure to choose chunk light tuna instead. Other fish with high levels of mercury are swordfish, mackerel, shark, and kingfish. Ocean salmon is the safest salmon to eat due to the fact that our fresh water streams and rivers are over eighty percent contaminated. Farm raised-salmon is also a health hazard. This is primarily due to the fact that farm-raised fish are given antibiotics and growth hormones, not to mention the fact that they swim in, and ingest their own waste because of the overcrowded conditions in their tanks. They have just enough of space to tread water. Their meat is actually chemically altered to give it a healthy pink color, which means more chemicals for us to consume.

An escalating number of chronic diseases are directly related to the environment in which we live. Medical researchers strongly believe that chemical exposure is responsible for environmental illnesses, such as asthma, multiple-chemical sensitivity (MCS), Parkinson's disease, non-Hodgkin's lymphoma, aplastic anemia, and various cancers. Immune system disorders are on the rise as well. Diseases like diabetes, multiple sclerosis, lupus, chronic fatigue syndrome, nervous-system disorders, and learning disorders (such as ADD, ADHD and autism) are now at an all-time high. Large contributors to immune-deficient diseases, including cancers of the reproductive system, are the many industrial chemicals known as endocrine disrupters. These chemicals possess estrogen-like compounds that mimic the female hormone estrogen.

It has been proven that women with high levels of estrogen have a greater risk of developing breast cancer. I am the co-founder and facilitator for A Woman's Circle of Hope, a breast-cancer support group. All but one member of the group was on some form of synthetic estrogen, ERT (estrogen replacement therapy) or birth control pills, prior to their diagnosis of breast cancer. Most of them were never told of the cancer risk involved in using HRT (hormone replacement therapy). They were told it was prescribed for controlling menopausal symptoms and for the prevention of osteoporosis. Millions of women are now paying dearly for the use of these synthetic chemicals. Environmental pollutants like the insecticide DDT, industrial PCBs, and petroleum by-products, all have estrogenic activity.

It is a known fact that PCBs have been linked to a depressed immune system, and a reduced fertility rate in males. PCBs have persisted in our environment, water and food, even though they were banned from use in 1976.

Cardiovascular Disease

I find it very interesting that in the early 1900s, the ten leading causes of death in the United States didn't include heart disease. Today, (as previously mentioned) heart disease is the number one killer for men and women. From birth, your chance of dying from cardiovascular disease is forty-seven percent. I am a firm believer that this number can be drastically reduced if more people were educated on disease prevention. The American diet is directly related to heart disease. Cardiovascular disease (CVD) is a general term that includes heart attack, stroke, and other heart and blood vessel disorders. There are over fifty million people walking around with CVD today. Unfortunately, many don't know they have it because they show no symptoms; and by the time symptoms occur, for some, it is too late. Each year over four hundred thousand people die in emergency rooms or on the way to the hospital. CVD kills more women than breast cancer and uterine cancer combined. It used to be thought of as a disease for men, but now over two hundred and fifty thousand women die annually from CVD. African-American women are at a higher risk than women of other ethnic backgrounds. Arteriosclerosis or hardening of the arteries is the most common cause of obstruction and is responsible for most of the deaths resulting from heart attacks. Risk factors for CVD are hypertension (high blood pressure), cigarette smoking, high cholesterol, obesity, and diabetes. With the exception of cigarette smoking, diet can prevent most of the other risk factors. High-fat diets have been linked to obesity, diabetes, hypertension, high cholesterol, heart disease and certain cancers.

Let's take a moment to discuss cholesterol. A total cholesterol level should be below 200 to be considered healthy, if it is between 200-239, then you are borderline problematic. For levels over 240, you are at high risk for major problems, such as plaque build-up in the arteries that can impede blood flow to the kidneys, brain, genitals, extremities, and the heart. High cholesterol is a primary cause of heart disease because it produces deposits in the arteries.

What exactly is cholesterol and why do we need it? Cholesterol is manufactured in the liver and transported through the bloodstream to travel to where it is needed. It is an essential part of every cell and is needed for brain and nerve function. Cholesterol is also the basis for the manufacture of sex hormones. It is a fatty substance and it latches onto molecules called lipoproteins to get around. Low-density lipoproteins (LDLs) are the major transporters of cholesterol in the blood and since LDLs encourage deposits of cholesterol in the arteries, it is considered the "bad cholesterol." I remember when I was learning about cholesterol it helped me to relate the word "lousy" to LDLs. This way I wouldn't forget which cholesterol was the bad cholesterol.

HDLs (high-density lipoproteins) are called the "good cholesterol" for the opposite reason. They escort the cholesterol that is not needed away from the cells and back to the liver, where it is broken down for removal from the body. When all goes well, the system remains in balance. If there is too much cholesterol for the HDLs to handle or if there isn't enough HDLs to do the job, then cholesterol can accumulate in the arteries forming plaque that will eventually lead to heart disease. A healthy HDL (good cholesterol) level is 60 mg or above. There are several healthy ways to reduce cholesterol levels without using prescription medications. There is an old folk remedy that has been successful for over seventy-five years. It is a drink prepared with eight ounces of distilled water, one teaspoon of raw honey and one teaspoon of apple cider vinegar with the mother (raw, unfiltered) in it (you can find these items at your health food store). This preparation is taken in the morning on an empty stomach and again before bed. Have patience and in about thirty days you will see impressive results. Apple pectin, oatmeal, and oat bran, aid in the elimination of cholesterol by escorting it out of the body.

Other foods to include in your diet for lowering cholesterol would be bananas, carrots, cold-water fish, dried beans, garlic, grapefruit, and olive oil. Reduce the amount of saturated fat and cholesterol in your diet. Saturated fats include all fats of animal origin, coconut oil, palm kernel oil and vegetable shortening. Avoid all hydrogenated fats like margarine, lard and butter, as well as products made with these fats. Start reading labels, it is the single most important thing you can do when choosing the foods you are about to consume. Know exactly what you are about to eat and whether it is good for your body or not. As I mentioned before, avoid any products that contain "hydrogenated" or "partially hydrogenated" oils. These are trans-fats and are very bad for you. Avoid heating oil to excessive heat this also produces harmful fats. Your best bet is olive oil for cooking.

Hypertension or high blood pressure is also a major factor in CVD. The heart pumps blood through the arteries and the blood presses against the walls of the blood vessels. In people with high blood pressure, this pressure is abnormally high. There are several factors involved to determine whether blood pressure is high, low, or normal. These factors are the output of the heart, the resistance to blood flow through the blood vessels, the volume of the blood, and blood distribution to various organs. If blood pressure is elevated then the heart must work harder to pump enough blood to all the tissues of the body. High blood pressure often leads to kidney failure, heart failure, and stroke. It is also associated with coronary heart disease, arteriosclerosis, kidney disorders, obesity, diabetes, hyperthyroidism, and adrenal tumors. Approximately thirty-five million people have high blood pressure and half of them are unaware that they are hypertensive.

Again, this was previously thought to be a man's disease, but women now equal the statistics of men. More women die from complications from this condition because women, and sometimes their physicians, often ignore, or fail to recognize the problem until it is too late. Hypertension is often referred to as the silent killer, due to the fact that symptoms don't usually appear until there are complications. This fact should be reason enough for people to stay on track with their annual physical exams and more importantly listen to your body for warning signs of hypertension. Some of these signs would be dizziness, headaches, sweating, rapid pulse, shortness of breath, and visual disturbances. If these symptoms should occur, get your blood pressure checked immediately. I am not a big fan of hypertensive medications, because of the additional complications and side effects that can occur from the use of these drugs. However, persistent high blood pressure can be a result of another underlying problem, such as kidney disease, hormonal abnormalities, or an inherited narrowing of the aorta, and may need additional treatment.

I believe that diet and lifestyle changes can reduce blood pressure without medications for many people. A diet most often recommended is a salt-free diet that is high in fiber and low in fat. Increasing plenty of fresh fruits and vegetables, such as apples, asparagus, bananas, broccoli, cabbage, cantaloupe, eggplant, garlic, green leafy vegetables, grapefruit, melons, peas, prunes, raisins, squash, and sweet potatoes will greatly improve your blood pressure levels. Fresh juices like carrot, beet, celery, current, cranberry, citrus, parsley, and spinach are particularly healthful. Eat grains like brown rice, buckwheat, millet and corn. Protein should come mostly from vegetables sources, grains, and legumes with added lean animal protein. Fat choices should include at least one tablespoon of flaxseed oil daily. Food to reduce or avoid all together would be animal fats, cheeses, aged meats, anchovies, avocados, chocolate, fava beans, pickled herring, and alcohol.

The FED Program will drastically lower cholesterol and high blood pressure, and will also help to stabilize blood sugar levels.

Cancer, on the Rise

Cancer has unfortunately become a household word. You hear about it every day whether from a newly diagnosed friend or family member, or in the media, such as in newspapers and magazines, and especially on television. It has become one of our greatest fears. Annual check-ups are a frightening experience, especially when additional tests are ordered for any suspicious areas and you are anxiously waiting for the results to be passed down. Do I have cancer or do I not? According to Patrick Quillin, the authoritative figure on *Beating Cancer With Nutrition,* we will all contract cancer at least six times in our lifetime. However, only forty-two percent of us will be diagnosed and end up in treatment. The deciding factor as to whether or not we will be diagnosed is dependant upon our immune status. The key to warding off cancer is to have a top-notch immune system, which can be acquired through proper nutrition. I will recommend numerous times in this book, that anyone battling cancer MUST purchase Patrick Quillin's book, Beating Cancer with Nutrition. It will change your life.

I haven't discussed thus far how I became acquainted with cancer. In November of 2000, my family received the devastating news that my sister, Stephanie, had been diagnosed with lobular breast cancer at thirty-five years of age. Having a sister with breast cancer, now added to the risk factor for the rest of the family, especially for myself and for my daughter. I immediately threw myself into learning mode, thirsting for as much information as I could get my hands on pertaining to how to prevent breast cancer. I joined a support group called, Bosom Buddies, and my journey began. What I was about to learn scared me to death, yet fueled me to learn more. I met some very courageous women and saw first hand what this dreaded disease could do to women of all ages, showing no prejudice to anyone.

My sister, thank God, did extremely well with her course of treatment and her prognosis was very good. Today she is a four-year survivor and we enthusiastically celebrate her survivorship every November. I eventually started volunteering as co-facilitator for the Bosom Buddies support group under the mentorship of Bobbi de'Cordova-Hanks, and found myself educating members on nutrition. I broadened my audience to include other cancer groups and businesses. Before I knew it I became a referred speaker on nutrition for the American Cancer Society.

Having seen, and continuing to see on a daily basis, the prevalence of cancer is what prompted me to write this book. I needed a tool that I could take out to groups to help them attain health and prevent disease. This book enables me to reach a broader audience. I pray that by educating the public on the many dangers that can be avoided and how to deal with those that can't, that together we can make a difference by beginning to win this war on cancer. I don't find it necessary to delve into the discouraging statistics of cancer. We all know how rapidly cancer is becoming of pandemic proportion. Now is the perfect time to take responsibility for your health by implementing the FED program for disease prevention, to further ensure that you won't become one of those devastating statistics.

The FED program is very closely related to a cancer prevention diet. Focus is on wholesome, nutritious foods and sugar is not one of them. It is a proven fact that cancer is fueled by glucose, meaning that sugar feeds cancer. It seems fairly simple then, that by eliminating sugar in the diet we can strengthen the odds of avoiding cancer. The FED program takes you back to basics detoxifying the body from sugar, caffeine, processed foods, and unhealthy fats, all of which suppress the immune system. It is said that the average American consumes approximately one hundred and seventy pounds of sugar annually including, over eight hundred doughnuts, sixty pounds of pastries (including cake and cookies), twenty-five gallons of ice cream, twenty-five pounds of candy, two hundred sticks of chewing gum and the average child today consumes one thousand eight hundred and twenty-five cans of soda.

Is there a correlation between these numbers and cancer? You bet, and these numbers just astound me! According to Patrick Quillin, forty-one percent of Americans don't consume fruit daily, eighty-two percent do not eat the power foods called cruciferous vegetables (broccoli, cauliflower, etc.), which are natures natural cancer fighters, and overall, over ninety-two percent of the American public does not consume the recommended daily allowance for vital vitamins and minerals. These facts, combined with the over consumption of sugar, is the equivalent of a train heading for derailment. The body is eventually going to break down and jump track.

Some of you may be wondering what's so bad about some of the food items listed above. Let me take a moment to enlighten those of you that feel soft drinks are a good choice of beverages. Most soft drinks are sweetened with a sweetener called high fructose corn syrup also known as HFCS. HFCS is a combination of corn syrup, which is a sweetener, and fructose, which is the natural sugar found in fruit. Either one of these alone would be utilized by the body as sugars to be used as energy. However, when combined, they form a structure that our body cannot recognize (sort of like a computer that can't read a program), and instead of using HFCS as a sugar/fuel source, it stores it as fat. Could this be why our younger generation is so overweight? Think of all the products that contain HFCS. Let's name a few, almost all cake and cookie snacks, pop tarts, cereals, most soft drinks, fruit drinks, fruit wrinkles or gummies, commercial applesauce, fruit cocktail, jams, fruit pops, ice cream, most candy products, ketchup, luncheon meats, puddings, pretzels, yogurt, snack bars, and even diet snacks. I think you get the picture.

If you're thinking you'll just purchase diet colas instead, you should know the facts first. Diet soft drinks are sweetened with aspartame, which is derived from the amino acids aspartate and phenylalanine. Aspartate and glutamate (as in MSG, mono-sodium glutamate) are called excitotoxins. They kill brain neurons, cause obesity and fertility problems, and have been known to cause the early onset of puberty in children. Excitotoxins have also been linked to lower thyroid hormone levels, and higher cortisol levels, as well as, to the prevalence of diabetes in the elderly. Are the pieces of the "food in correlation to disease"' puzzle beginning to fit? It's a wonder that any of us have any brain cells left after the many years of abuse from these products. I was a big diet beverage drinker of products containing aspartame and I am sure most of you dieters were too. Well, now you know better. I said it before and you'll most certainly hear it again, "now is the perfect time to implement change beginning with your diet." There are many other alternative beverages for you to consume instead of soft drinks. This change will not only benefit you it will affect your entire family. I recently read that the average child in America consumes over sixty-four ounces of soft drinks daily. I honestly believe that this number reflects the astronomical increase in ADD and ADHD in children.

Chapter Three

The Importance of Supplementation

Recent studies have proven how beneficial vitamins, minerals and other supplements can be in improving your overall health and in protecting you from heart disease, diabetes, cancer and other chronic diseases. With this in mind I have carefully chosen the supplements for the FED program. The recommended supplements will work synergistically (working together) with the food choices on the program to obtain optimal health. Most of us are at a quandary when it comes to supplements. For example, questions arise such as the following:

1. Should I take a multivitamin; and if so, what brand should I take?

2. How much is enough; and can too much be dangerous?

3. Is it better to take single nutrients or combinations?

Because of the saturation of supplements on the market today, I have taken the liberty to tell you exactly which supplements to take. All multivitamins are not equal. Every single one is different from the next. I researched and cross-referenced my choices for supplements many times over to ensure that I chose the right ones for this program. As I outline the supplements you will be taking, I will also educate you on the many aspects of supplements to help you better understand the importance of supplementation.

With regard to whether or not to take a multivitamin, the answer is simply, yes! In this day and age, with air pollution, water pollution and other environmental toxins, I feel everyone can benefit from at least a good quality multivitamin. With all the additives, antibiotics, growth hormones and artificial coloring in the food we eat, our body constantly has to filter out toxins, thus taxing the liver. Another problem for the liver is the fact that vitamins are concentrated; and if you don't drink a full glass of water when taking your multi, they too can overburden the liver. Water actually enhances their absorption. The liver is the gatekeeper for all nutrients. It designates their destination within the body. The FED program is designed to support this overworked organ; and a good multivitamin will do just that.

As far as which brands you should purchase, try to stay away from generic, no name, and cheap brands. You truly get what you pay for. Try brands that are reputable and meet recommended daily allowances (RDA) and daily values (DV) from the National Academy of Sciences' U.S. Food and Nutrition board. For example, calcium and magnesium should be at a two to one ratio, however, those numbers can be reversed based on an individual's needs. Copper and zinc's daily value should be pretty equal because if zinc values are elevated, it can impair the absorption of copper. Daily values are for adults and children over four years of age, at least for now. This RDA guideline was implemented over forty years ago by the National Academy of Sciences' U.S. Food and Nutrition board, and was created with the healthy person in mind. Most nutritionists agree that these values are extremely low and that everyone couldn't possibly fit into one category when it comes to nutrients; and the RDA guideline implies that everyone is the same and has the same nutritional needs. This is one more reason why a sound diet is of vital importance. I wonder how a four year old and a two hundred-pound man can have the same requirements for nutrients!

Some abbreviations that are important to know are as follows:

1. mg. = milligram.

2. mcg. = microgram.

3. I.U. = international units.

International units are how fat-soluble vitamins, such as A, D, E, and K are measured. These vitamins must be taken prior to or with a meal containing fat. Water-soluble vitamins can be taken with or after the meal. Vitamins absorb better when taken with food. I personally recommend taking them at the end of a meal, so you can take them with at least eight ounces water. Consuming water with your meal can impede digestion, due to the fact that water will dilute enzymes and digestive juices.

It is also important to check the expiration date on the bottom of the bottle or packaging, as they will begin to lose potency after the expiration date. You should try to use the organic or natural form of vitamins as they are more easily absorbed and easier on the body. Folate is the natural form and folic acid is synthetic, d-alpha tocopherol is natural and dl-alpha tocopherol is synthetic, ferrous sulfate is the synthetic form of iron and if taken regularly (along with certain medications) can cause health problems. Ferrous gluconate, citrate and fumerate are the natural preferred forms of iron. Studies have proven that an excess amount of vitamins and minerals can produce the same symptoms as deficiencies. Proper balance is very important. There are actually very few vitamins and minerals that can be toxic if taken in excess, however, there are plenty of contraindications between supplements and medications and certain medical conditions. For example, it is advised not to exceed 10,000 IU of vitamin A if you are pregnant or have liver disease; and cod liver oil when taken as a supplement, is a definite contraindication for liver ailments. Those with liver problems also need to use niacin B3 with caution, not to exceed 500 mg. daily, although there is a safer form available called inositol hexaniacinate, and this does not affect the liver. Do not exceed more than 100 mg. of zinc daily because it can depress the immune system. These are just a few examples of how taking supplements without researching them first can be hazardous. It is strongly advised to seek the advice of a professional, especially if you are on medications, before you start taking supplements. Most contraindications or interactions are not serious, but some can be fatal. With all of this in mind, let us begin to delve into the individual supplements for the FED program.

Multivitamin

A multi vitamin and mineral supplement is a very important part of the FED program. It is the added insurance we need to ensure that we get the required amount of nutrients. The foods you will be consuming on this program will give you most of the nutrients that the body requires, however, many of us don't have the best digestive tract and digestion may be impeded for a number of reasons. Therefore, a good performance multi is recommended. There is a wealth of information available to you from individual supplement manufacturers. Do your homework and research the multi of your choice. I have taken the liberty to list a few of these companies in the reference section of this book.

When purchasing a multi vitamin try to choose a multi that contains these important vitamins and minerals: vitamins A, C, D, E, K, all the Bs including folic acid and biotin (to normalize fat metabolism and utilization and reduce blood sugar levels); choline (supports the liver and kidneys, and is needed for the emulsification of fats and cholesterol, and is referred to as the memory vitamin); calcium (bone health);, magnesium (considered the anti-stress mineral, prevents heart disease, kidney stones, and lowers blood pressure); iodine (for thyroid function); zinc (improves immune function); copper; selenium (prevents cardiovascular disease, certain cancers, stimulates immune function, speeds healing and recovery time, helpful in treating skin conditions, and reduces menopausal symptoms); manganese (anti-inflammatory properties, aids glucose metabolism, and may prevent the proliferation of cancer cells); chromium (beneficial in the treatment of hypoglycemia and diabetes, lowers cholesterol and triglycerides, and may prevent heart disease); molybdenum (may help prevent anemia, may reduce uric acid formation, may prevent certain cancers, and protects against the ill effects of sufites); and zinc.

The following powerful supplements can also be beneficial and depending on the product you choose they may already be included: Bee pollen (antimicrobial, useful for fatigue, depression, certain cancers, and colon disorders, also beneficial for allergy suffers because it strengthens immune function, however, avoid if you have an allergy to bee pollen) citrus bioflavonoids, cranberry concentrate (protects against urinary and bladder infections, is a diuretic, has anticancer properties, and is a good source of vitamin C), para-aminobenzoic acid PABA (protects our skin against harmful rays of the sun thus preventing skin cancer), royal jelly (useful against bronchial asthma, liver disease, panceatitis, kidney disease, ulcers of the stomach, bone fractures, skin disorders, and strengthens immune function), silica, boron, red raspberry leaves (good for reproductive health, bones, nails, teeth, and skin, menopausal and PMS symptoms), lutein (anti-cancer agent), and inositol (cancer fighter, may prevent heart, kidney and liver disease, lowers cholesterol, helps to maintain immune integrity during cancer treatment).

As you can see a good supplement can offer many beneficial properties pertaining to disease prevention. Be sure to check the proper dosing as most vitamins require two caplets/capsules per dose. Also be aware of added preservatives, colorants, and fillers. It truly pays to research new products before purchasing them. I did an experiment on several name brand vitamins. This involved placing the vitamins in a beaker of hydrochloric acid to see if they would disintegrate and how long they took to dissolve. I was shocked to discover that a few of them took forever to dissolve and that some didn't dissolve at all. This gave me a great indication as to how they would perform in our bodies.

You should also be aware if the company refuses to disclose certain information pertaining to a product. For example a client of mine asked me to see what I could find out about sea silver. He had heard great things about it and was very impressed with their infomercial. I approached the company and requested the nutritional breakdown of their product and was refused this information. They told me it was a "proprietary blend" and that should suffice. I immediately reported to my client that I would not recommend anything that wasn't one hundred percent on the up and up. If a company refuses to give out detailed information about their product, then I draw the conclusion that they are either hiding something, or are involved in false advertising. It is too easy to get caught up in the hype and hoopla of a new product, especially, if it is over-saturated within the market. We would all love that quick fix, cure-all, magic pill that would make us feel great. But I will tell you now that this product does NOT exist. You can only achieve this by consuming the proper foods that the body needs to thrive. I have personally found that most illnesses result from malabsorption syndrome, which is the failure to absorb nutrients. A single nutrient depletion can cause all kinds of problems, within the body, over a period of time. This is why I find it extremely important to take a good, highly absorbable multi-vitamin mineral supplement.

As I mentioned earlier, if you are unclear as to which supplement is right for you, then please refer to the reference section of this book or speak to your health care professional to recommend a good supplement for you.

Flaxseed Oil

Flaxseed oil has a wealth of medicinal properties. It has 6200 mg. of omega 3, 1810 mg. of omega 6, and 2040 mg. of omega 9 per tablespoon. It contains 110 calories and 10 grams of healthy fats, and only one gram of saturated fat per tablespoon. The many health benefits include: protection against heart disease, strokes, diabetes, anticarcinogenic activity against tumors, aids in the treatment of arthritis, asthma, inflammatory disease, premenstrual syndrome, multiple sclerosis, and helps to normalize blood sugar. Flaxseed also aids in fat metabolism, increases vitality, improves immune function, and protects against cold weather resistance. Other health benefits associated with flaxseed are, increased function of the adrenals, reproductive system, and brain. It is also used to improve certain psychiatric behavior disorders.

Flaxseed has a special fiber called lignin, which converts to lignans in our body, which help to improve immunity and has anticancer, antifungal, and antiviral properties. Flax has been used to improve menopausal symptoms, reduce cholesterol and triglyceride levels, treat burns and external wounds, and it can even sooth coughs. If there were any questions as to why I picked this particular fat and supplement for the FED program, I hope flaxseed oil's many attributes will speak for themselves. The benefits from consuming flaxseed oil are endless. All the sources I read on this medicinal oil state that you should be able to see benefits after two to three months of use. Make sure you consume one tablespoon of flaxseed oil daily and I strongly encourage you to continue this beneficial supplement even after the completion of this program.

Evening Primrose or Black Current Oil

Evening Primrose oil contains approximately ten percent of gamma-linolenic acid, also referred to as GLA and also has a wealth of medicinal benefits such as, prevents hardening of the arteries, heart disease, multiple sclerosis, reduces premenstrual syndrome and menopausal symptoms, and high blood pressure. It can relieve pain, inflammation, treat eczema and other skin disorders, and is a muscle relaxant. Caution should be exercised for women with breast cancer, especially if the cancer is estrogen positive, because Evening Primrose oil promotes the production of estrogen. Black current oil, which shares similar properties as Evening Primrose (except for the estrogen factor), would be the supplement for you.

Lecithin Granules

Lecithin (also called phosphatidylcholine), is an important form of fat called phospholipids. Lecithin is found in all animals and plant products, including: cabbage, cauliflower, caviar, eggs, garbonzo beans, green beans, lentils, organ meats, seed/nuts, soy lecithin, soybeans, and split peas. Lecithin is the major source of choline; however, lecithin must be present in the body before choline synthesis can occur. Those that are taking niacin for the treatment of high serum cholesterol and triglycerides need to take choline or lecithin supplements. Lecithin's many benefits are: it protects against damage to cells by oxidation, prevents heart disease, supports the liver, and lowers cholesterol. Lecithin has also been used for, arteriosclerosis, improving brain function, bipolar depression disorder, energy levels and fat metabolism, aids those suffering from chronic fatigue syndrome, aids, herpes, and other immune disorders. Lecithin actually works as a general detoxifier for the body by decongesting the liver of excess fats.

I happen to enjoy the taste of lecithin and consume it daily for many of these reasons. Lecithin was a very popular supplement in the '70s and is once again regaining its popularity. You can purchase it in two forms, capsules or granules. I prefer lecithin granules. They come in plain or apple cinnamon flavor. They can be mixed into smoothies, sprinkled in yogurt, or taken straight by the tablespoon, which is my favorite way to take lecithin and I usually will take my fat soluble vitamins along with it, as well. Lecithin is good for all ages, especially the aged, or anyone suffering from cognitive malfunction (this is my technical term for "forgetting"). I call lecithin my brain-food supplement.

Probiotics

Probiotics find their way into every one of my disease prevention protocols. I feel they can benefit anyone taking them. Probiotics are beneficial bacteria that are found in the digestive tract. They are of vital importance when it comes to proper digestion. They perform a number of tasks including, preventing yeast overgrowth, and synthesizing certain B vitamins and vitamin K.

The type of probiotic that you are probably most familiar with is

Lactobacillus Acidophilus– and yes, it is found in yogurt. You can also find it in kefir, and other fermented foods. According to Phyllis A. Balch, CNC, a healthy colon should contain approximately eighty-five percent lactobacilli and fifteen percent coliform bacteria, however, the typical bacteria within the colon today is actually the opposite. This causes all sorts of health problems such as, bloating, gas, toxicity, constipation, and most importantly malabsorption of nutrients. The use of probiotics can alleviate many of these problems by bringing the intestinal flora back into balance.

Probiotic literally means "for life." There are many strains of beneficial bacteria other then acidophilus, however, the most recognized and used in probiotic supplements are Lactobacillus acidophilus, which is beneficial to the small intestine and Lactobacillus Bifidis, for the large intestine or colon. Probiotics come in various forms. They come in capsules, powders, tablets, and liquids. Acidophilus is actually touted as an antibiotic, as well. This is because acidophilus (friendly bacteria) creates an environment within the intestines that is not conducive to many pathogens: bacterial, viral and of other origin.

Yogurt can be consumed by people with lactose intolerance because of a deficiency of the lactase enzyme. Bacteria change or ferment the lactose sugar and produce lactic acid. There have been health claims made by some people that yogurt actually settles an upset stomach, is great for intestinal gas, and even helps soothe inflammatory problems of the stomach. Many probiotic users, such as myself, also swear that they improve immune function, lessen the effects of allergies, and reduces the risk for certain cancers, specifically of the colon, stomach, and colorectal. If you are going to consume yogurt I recommend only purchasing organic brands. I elaborate on the reasons why in the next chapter.

A friend of mine, Valerie Miles, MD, a holistic pediatrician, is also an advocate of probiotics. She has recommended it to several of my clients who have children with recurrent ear infections, and it amazes me every time when I hear the feedback of praise from these parents, many of them wishing they'd known about probiotics years ago. There is a wonderful product by Natrens called Life Start. Life Start is a probiotic that is specially formulated for infants. It is recommended for many babies, particularly those that were not breast fed. Formulas can be very hard on a baby's digestive system. Life Start gives the digestive tract the beneficial bacteria it needs aiding in the digestion process. Probiotics will also improve your child's immune function.

Digestive Enzymes

This powerful digestive aid is also a highly recommended supplement in my practice. In this day and age we can all stand to have a little digestive help. One of the many problems with digestion begins in the mouth with improper chewing habits, which I have already addressed in Chapter One. If we were to improve upon our chewing, we would drastically cut down on the wear and tear of our digestive system; and in return we would have a better absorption rate for nutrients. With the fast-paced lives we lead, this isn't always possible and we are unfortunately eating on the run more than we should. If you fall into this category, then you are definitely a candidate for digestive enzymes.

Digestive enzymes are secreted all through the digestive tract. They break down foods enabling the food to absorb into the bloodstream. The three main categories for digestive enzymes are: amylase, protease, and lipase. Amylase is an enzyme that breaks down carbohydrates and is found in saliva, pancreatic and intestinal juices. There are several different types of amylase, such as lactase breaks down lactose (milk sugar), sucrase breaks down the sugar called sucrose (cane or beet sugar) and maltase breaks down maltose (malt sugar). Protease, on the other hand, breaks down protein. Protease is found in the stomach, intestinal, and pancreatic juices, and of course lipase is responsible for the breakdown of fat, and can be found in the stomach and pancreatic juices, as well as in foods that contain fat.

Most of the commercial products for digestive enzymes come from animal sources and plant sources. One of the sources comes from animal enzymes like pancreatin and pepsin, which aid in digestion once the food has entered into the lower stomach. Another form of digestive enzyme is made from the enzyme of aspergillus, which is a fungus. These enzymes begin working in the upper stomach. Each of these products was created to aid digestion and absorption of nutrients, especially that of protein. There is a disorder called, "Leaky Gut Syndrome," which is caused from the inability to breakdown protein. This occurs from undigested protein particles that make their way into the bloodstream through the intestinal wall, along with other nutrients. By using the proper digestive enzymes called proteolytic enzymes, which break down protein, you can help to prevent this problem. Two popular plant food enzymes called bromelain and papain, come from pineapple and papaya, both are proteolytic enzymes. They come in chewable forms and are taken after a meal containing protein. They are a delicious way to aid digestion; and children love them too.

Digestive enzymes are available in tablet, capsule, liquid and powder form. Many of them are available in combination form. The one I recommend is a combo form called Digest by Enzymedica, and contains: Amylase, protease, lipase, cellulase, lactase, alpha-galactosidase, malt diatase, invertase, pectinase, and even contains some probiotics. I have found that this digestive enzyme covers it all. The recommended dosage is one capsule with every meal; however, everyone is different and has different needs. Things to consider are, how much food was consumed at the meal, was alcohol included (alcohol slows down digestion and inhibits certain enzymic reactions), and the health of the individual, especially the efficacy of their digestive system. I usually take one a day with my heaviest protein meal.

Enzymes can also be found in other plant food sources such as: bananas, avocados, mangoes, and apples. Sprouts are one of the richest sources for enzymes. Heat destroys most enzymes; therefore, eating these foods raw will insure that you retain the enzymes. Alternately, taking digestive enzyme supplements will greatly help to prevent the depletion of the body's enzymes; thus reducing stress on the digestive system and the body as a whole.

This covers the recommended supplements for the FED program; however, there are a few supplements that I'd like to inform you about for added disease prevention. These four phenomenal antioxidant-supplements work synergistically (working together), for optimum protection. They are vitamins A, C, E, and selenium. For example: when vitamin E has mopped up a reactive oxygen species, the vitamin E is also oxidized. This oxidized vitamin E must then be turned back to its' active form and that is where vitamin C comes to the rescue, turning vitamin E back into its active form. All four of these antioxidants work in this manner. Let's take a look at these four supplements individually.

A-C-E-S for Prevention

I highly recommend adding these powerful mega vitamins: vitamins A, C, and E, and the mineral Selenium, to your diet for disease prevention.

Vitamin A is a fat-soluble vitamin and needs to be taken with a meal containing fat. Vitamin A prevents night blindness, and other eye ailments, enhances immunity, aids in the healing of gastrointestinal ulcers, is important in the formation of bones and teeth, aids in fat storage, and protects against colds, flu, and infections of the kidneys, bladder, lungs, and mucous membranes. As an antioxidant, it helps protect the cells against cancer and other diseases. Certain symptoms such as, dry hair, dry skin, dry eyes, poor growth, night blindness, infections of the ears, insomnia, fatigue, reproductive difficulties, sinusitis, frequent infections, and weight loss may indicate a deficiency in vitamin A.

Vitamin A is found in animal livers, apricots, asparagus, beet greens, broccoli, cantaloupe, carrots, collards, dandelion greens, dulse, fish liver and fish liver oil, garlic, kale, mustard greens, papayas, pumpkin, peaches, red peppers, spinach, spirulina, sweet potatoes, swiss chard, turnip greens, watercress, and yellow squash. It is also found in abundance in herbs.

Note: Animal sources of vitamin A are up to six times as strong as vegetable sources.

Vitamin C is a one of the most powerful antioxidants and is required for over three hundred metabolic functions within the body. Some of these functions include: the growth and repair of tissue, the functioning of the adrenals and the production of anti-stress hormones and interferon, which is an important immune system protein. There is documented research that proves its' efficacy for the reduction of asthmatic symptoms, protection against chronic diseases like cancer and cardiovascular disease, fighting off bacterial and viral infections, as well as preventing the formation of cataracts. Vitamin C also enhances immunity, increases the absorption of iron, and aids in the elimination of toxic substances, such as heavy metals, and promotes the healing of burns and wounds.

Vitamin C works synergistically with vitamins A (beta carotene) and E. Together these vitamins reinforce and extend each other's antioxidant capabilities. Vitamin C is called an essential vitamin because the body does not produce it and it has to be obtained through diet. Some valuable food sources for Vitamin C include: berries, citrus, green leafy vegetables, asparagus, avocados, beet greens, black currents, broccoli, brussels sprouts, cantaloupe, dulse, onions, papaya, green peas, peppers, pineapple, persimmons, radishes, and one of the highest sources is from kiwi. It is also found in abundance among herbs.

There are several factors that can cause serious depletions of vitamin C within the body, such as the use of alcohol, antidepressants, analgesics, anticoagulants, oral contraceptives, steroids and smoking.

Vitamin C comes in many forms and should be consumed in divided doses, two to three times daily. Ester C is a very effective form of vitamin C because it enters the bloodstream up to four times faster than other forms. It also moves into blood cells and tissue faster and more effectively while lasting longer within the body. I take 2000 mg. daily for the above health benefits.

Vitamin E is of vital importance in the prevention of diseases such as cancer and heart disease. It has long been known for improving circulation, promoting normal blood clotting and healing, reducing blood pressure, premenstrual symptoms, and fibrocystic breast disease. Vitamin E also enhances reproduction, prevents cataracts, and has been shown to slow the progression of Alzheimer's disease. There are studies proving the efficacy of vitamin E in protecting us from over eighty diseases.

There are several symptoms of deficiency including, infertility, menstruation problems, spontaneous abortion, uterine degeneration, neuromuscular impairment and the shortened lifespan of red blood cells. Low levels of E have been linked to cancers of the breast and colon. Vitamin E needs other nutrients, such as zinc in order to maintain levels in the blood. It also needs vitamin C to aid its war against free radicals, as I mentioned earlier. Vitamin E should never be taken with iron, take them separately at different times of the day. Inorganic forms of iron, such as ferrous sulfate will destroy vitamin E whereas, organic forms won't.

Vitamin E can be found in many food sources like, dark green leafy vegetables, legumes, nuts, seeds, whole grains, dulse, eggs, kelp, desiccated liver, milk, oatmeal, organ meats, soybeans, sweet potatoes, watercress, wheat, and wheat germ. Natural sources should always be chosen over synthetic forms of vitamin E. The natural form is more available for use by the body then the synthetic version. The synthetic form is listed as dl-alpha-tocopherol, so be sure to read labels.

Selenium is a vital antioxidant as well, especially when combined with vitamin E. It protects our immune system by inhibiting the formation of free radicals. Selenium is also important in the role of regulating the effects of thyroid hormone on fat metabolism and protects against several forms of cancer including, lung, prostate, and colorectal by acting as a preventative against the formation of tumors. Selenium and vitamin E work hard together, to help support the liver, and heart.

Those suffering from a deficiency of selenium would experience exhaustion, stunted growth, high cholesterol levels, recurrent infections, problems affecting the liver and pancreas, and fertility problems. All my sources go back and forth on the varying levels of toxicity for this trace mineral. The safe recommended dosage is 100-200 mcg. daily. Excessive levels of selenium can cause arthritis, brittle hair and nails, bad breath, gastrointestinal disorders, irritability, liver and kidney problems, jaundice, and a metallic taste in your mouth.

Selenium can be found in meat and grains, brazil nuts, Brewer's yeast, broccoli, brown rice, chicken, dairy products, dulse, garlic, kelp, liver, onions, molasses, seafood, vegetables, wheat grass, wheat germ; and is also found in many beneficial herbs.

I have found that many of my clients benefit by adding in these four vital supplements. When I lecture on the importance of supplementation, I use the phrase, "A-C-E-S for Optimal Health." This makes it easier to remember vitamins A, C, E, and selenium. In conclusion, I hope you now realize the importance of taking these beneficial supplements, along with consuming a sound diet to achieve optimum health.

Drug Contraindications

I mentioned earlier that I would include information on drug, food, and supplement interactions. First of all, a contraindication is any symptom or circumstance that makes treatment with a drug or device unsafe or inappropriate. I must stress that this is a very important part of the FED program. If you are taking pharmaceutical drugs and supplements it is imperative to know if there are any contraindications between the two. It is estimated that over five hundred thousand people die annually from taking pharmaceutical drugs properly in the Unites States. Notice I said "properly" not improperly. They are dying because of the predictable side-effects of prescription drugs, according to Phyllis Balch, CNC. Thousands more die from the unpredictable side-affects of drugs and unfortunately, from the drug-to-drug contraindications. I must also say that in the United States there are very few deaths annually from supplements and herbal remedies combined. That is a big difference in statistics.

Among my clients who attend my lectures, I have found numerous problems with the medications they were taking. Some had been taking these medications for years not knowing the dangers they have been avoiding. For example, there is a woman in one of my FED groups that has been taking acid inhibitors for over eight years. She was just recently told that her iron stores are dangerously low. Her doctor wanted to put her on synthetic iron. Let's think about this for a moment. In order to absorb iron you need a sufficient amount of hydrochloric acid in your stomach. If you are taking an acid inhibitor, which inhibits the production of hydrochloric acid, then how do you think your body is going to absorb iron? I have found this same situation in several other clients who have been taking acid blockers or inhibitors for years - sometimes several times a day. One of these clients is my mother, Mary Lou Leist. My mother's experience with this problem is what prompted me to investigate this matter further. Her doctors didn't make the correlation between the acid blocker and the iron, however, after stopping the acid blocker and taking a natural source of supplemental iron, her iron stores slowly began to rise. A change in diet also helped her acid reflux problem. Some proton-pump-inhibitors (acid blockers) also cause a deficiency of beta-carotene, B-12, folic acid, and copper. This is just one class of drugs. And it is sad to say that there are many more that cause even greater problems, some resulting in death.

A good rule of thumb that will help you is, if you are taking a prescription drug for certain ailments never take a supplement or herbal remedy that does the same thing. For example, if you are taking cholesterol medication (statins) you wouldn't want to take red yeast rice, which also lowers cholesterol levels, because this would be considered an adverse interaction and can cause problems. The red yeast rice contains HMG-CoA reductase inhibitors, the same properties that the prescription drug contains. Take one or the other. Niacin (B3) is also contraindicative to this class of medicine when taken in high doses and can be very dangerous causing myopathy (muscle disorders). By the way, a high-fiber diet will decrease the effect of statins and also cause the depletion of Co Q10. It is recommended that you take the herb 'milk thistle' to support the liver while taking these drugs, due to the fact that cholesterol-lowering drugs cause liver toxicity. I would also like to mention the contraindication between taking diuretic medications and consuming unsweetened cranberry juice.

I have had a few clients that are taking diuretics for water retention; and after a couple of days on the FED program, their ankles started swelling. I immediately took them off the cranberry juice, instructing them to drink only water with lemon or lime, and within a few days the swelling had gone down considerably. Cranberry is also a diuretic and is a contraindication to diuretic medications. You should always check with your pharmacist, before taking a new medication, for any contraindications or adverse reactions.

Never think for a moment, that just because your doctor prescribes a drug for you, that the drug is safe. I personally have lost a loved one due to the wrong treatment and medications being administered, while in the hospital. Protect yourself and your family by educating yourself on the many dangers of pharmaceutical drugs and their interactions. One of my favorite quotes comes from Thomas Edison and is filled with hope for our future. He stated that, "The doctor of the future will give no medicine, but will interest his patients in the care of the human frame, in diet, and in the prevention of disease."

Testimonial

MARY LOU

I am a sixty-four-year-old female who has had a weight problem for most of my life. Over the past twenty years my health began to deteriorate and I was prescribed several medications that promote weight gain. As a result of this and several health-related factors, there was a substantial gain in weight. I soon became dependent on large amounts of medications including Axid, Darvocet, Motrin, Percocet, and synthetic iron for iron deficiency. Jennifer introduced me to the FED program and I was gradually able to come off some of the medications, which was quite an accomplishment considering the number of years I was dependent on these medications. I am now taking a natural iron supplement; and I am happy to say that my iron stores are replenishing for the first time in four years. I have lost approximately forty-two pounds in four months, as well as several inches in my body measurements. My high blood pressure is also now under control. I am deeply grateful to Jennifer for her dedication and perseverance of the FED program.

Chapter Four

You Are What You Eat, Foods For The FED Program

"You are what you eat" is the guiding principle behind The Fat Elimination and Detox Program (FED). FED is a healthy, wholesome way to lose weight safely and effectively. This program is based on an individual basis and is based on your basal metabolic rate (BMR) and overall health status. As a nutritionist, I will teach you how to eat for optimum health and explain how the foods you consume can prevent diseases like heart disease, cancer, and other chronic diseases, while losing weight for long-term health benefits. The FED program consists of eight weeks that are broken down into four segments.

The first segment represents the first two weeks of the program. The average weight loss during this segment is six to fourteen pounds, depending on individual circumstances. There are certain obstacles that may hinder weight loss, such as the usage of pharmaceutical drugs and treatments; and weight loss may be slower for those with disabilities or chronic disease. I have also found that pre-menopausal women will have a temporary set point, also called a plateau, during certain times of their cycle. This is a normal response in the body and should not induce discouragement.

FED was designed to educate people on disease prevention, while implementing a "complete" weight-loss program. I personally deal with chronic disease on a day-to-day basis in my practice, and was determined to develop a program that would efficiently shed the pounds, while nourishing and protecting the body. With these criteria in mind, I devised a program that would detoxify and support the entire body, as excess weight is lost, while saving wear and tear on the liver and kidneys, which greatly suffer under other weight-loss plans. The liver is the master organ for fat metabolism; if the liver isn't functioning properly, then weight loss will be hindered.

The first few weeks of the program do not allow for dairy or wheat. The FED program is not suitable for vegetarians because of the animal protein requirements. However, vegetarians that are piscopolarians (vegetarians that consume fish and poultry) can do quite nicely with this program. Weeks one and two are identical in structure and consist of basic organic food choices. I can't stress the word 'organic' enough. Pesticides and herbicides, antibiotics and growth hormones, are destructive to our health, as you have read in the previous chapters. However, consuming organic food during this program will seriously improve your health status by giving your body and vital organs a much needed break.

Organic foods can be costly, especially for a large family. Most of the food you will be purchasing is produce, which is one of the most important foods on this program. If purchasing organic produce is an issue, there are two solutions that will help you. The first is to purchase regular commercial produce, but also buy a good vegetable/fruit wash. The one I use is called "A Fruit and Veggie Wash," plain and simple, and can be purchased for just a few dollars. Spray the fruit or vegetables, then rub gently and rinse thoroughly. The other option is to make a wash using one gallon of clean cool water, then adding half to one teaspoon of Clorox, better known as bleach. Allow the fruit/vegetables to soak for twenty to thirty minutes then rinse thoroughly, pat dry and store in containers. Adding a dry paper towel to the container will lengthen the life of the fruit or vegetables. Fruits and vegetables are the staple of this program, making up approximately fifty percent of the food you'll be eating, so let me begin by educating you on the many benefits of fruit.

Fruit

Fruit is considered nature's most perfect food, ready made for us right from the plant it grows on. It is packed full of phytonutrients, also called phytochemicals, which are nutrients or chemicals found in plant foods. Phytonutrients have three functions within the body. First and foremost, they act as antioxidants, protecting us from the ravages of free radicals. Free radicals are molecules that have lost an electron, for numerous reasons, that seek out healthy molecules to steal their electron. This in turn transforms those healthy molecules into free radicals as well, and so on, and so on, until we have developed serious health problems. Phytonutrients create a protective force field around healthy cells, and give free radicals electrons to set them straight. They also help to regulate hormones, keeping hormone levels in balance, which is imperative for staving off disease. Certain phytonutrients can guard against viruses and bacteria, as well. Their third claim to fame is toxin elimination. Phytonutrients accomplish this by detoxifying carcinogens, which are cancer-causing chemicals and escorting them out of the body. There are literally hundreds of phytonutrients and they are all found in plant foods. By consuming fruits and vegetables, as directed on the FED program, you will be rewarded all of these health benefits.

Some of the fruits you will be eating during the first two weeks of the program are high in fiber and low on the glycemic index, such as berries, apples, pears, lemons, limes, peaches, apricots, cherries, and grapefruit. The glycemic index was devised to show how quickly a carbohydrate food assimilates into the blood, as compared to glucose, which is 99 on the index. Certain fruits like dried dates, watermelon, cantaloupe, pineapple, raisins, bananas, and mangoes, are not allowed the first few weeks on the program because of their high sugar content, however they will be added back in (in moderation) later on. There are three fruit choices daily.

As I mentioned previously sugar feeds cancer. Sugar also suppresses immune function. If we look back over the past fifty to sixty years, we would see that the food industry's inception of high-sugar foods correlates with the steady rise in cancer. For this very reason, I have eliminated high-glycemic foods from the FED program. Your fruit choices will be your source for fiber and valuable vitamins and minerals; and even though they are still a simple carbohydrate (sugar), called fructose, they are acceptable because of their many health benefits. They will serve the purpose of three snacks throughout the day and evening. I eat at least one apple a day with cinnamon to help regulate blood sugar levels. You will be given a more in-depth list in the next chapter when you begin the program.

Vegetables

Vegetables are an equally impressive component of the FED program when compared to fruit. Vital phytonutrients will aid us in our healing, detoxification, and protection from all health woes. Vegetables and fruits are often referred to as "power foods" because of their many medicinal properties. Phytonutrients, for example, the allylic sulfides, which are onions and garlic, are powerful warriors for fighting viral, bacterial, and fungal infections. They also aid in detoxifying the liver, lowering cholesterol, fat and blood sugar levels, and to top it off, protect us from certain cancers. Flavonoids, such as kale, endive, and broccoli, protect us from a plethora of health problems like heart disease, cancer, blood clots, ulcers, tumors, viruses, and cataracts. Carotenoids, work as a preventative for breast, prostate, lung, colorectal, and uterine cancers, arteriosclerosis, heart disease and stoke, and are found in carrots, spinach, broccoli, and most yellow, orange, and red vegetables and fruits. Glucosinolates are a potent form of phytonutrients that are found in cauliflower, broccoli, cabbage, bok choy, and brussels sprouts. They activate enzymes that detoxify the liver, protect us from most cancers, regulate white blood cells, thus boosting immune function, and block enzymes that promote tumor growth. These are just a few of the many phytonutrients and their many purposes. You will learn more about individual foods when you begin the program. You will be consuming a lot of vegetables on the FED program to ensure that you get all of these health benefits. Vegetables are probably the most crucial aspect for the prevention and detoxification process.

The vegetables that are acceptable during the first two weeks of the program include: peppers, cucumbers, mushrooms, sprouts (both clover and alfalfa), radishes, tomatoes, lettuce, carrots, green beans, daikon, onion, garlic, cabbage, broccoli, brussels sprouts, chard, collard greens, leeks, summer squash, zucchini, cauliflower, water chestnuts, jicama, spinach, green beans, artichokes, avocado, and turnips. Your vegetable serving size will average one cup per serving, however, you must consume eight to ten servings daily if you are on the low BMR program (1200-1600 calories), and ten to twelve servings daily if you are on the higher BMR program (1600-2000 calories) and ten to fourteen cups for the highest BMR program (2000-2400 calories). I know that sounds like a lot of vegetables, but keep in mind that an average size salad is about four to six cups of vegetables. You can then have a cup during the day of celery, fennel, or one of my favorites, sliced Napa cabbage as additional snacks. If you eat cabbage raw, you'll find it is very sweet for a vegetable, without having a glycemic index rating at all. For your evening meal, have two more cups of vegetables and that covers your quota for the day. If you are not fond of vegetables, I think there is no time like the present to change your mindset about this highly-medicinal food group. Not consuming vegetables is NOT an option on the FED program. Fruits and vegetables make up the carbohydrate portion of the FED program. The daily percentage for carbohydrates is fifty percent.

Grains

Grains are not allowed on the FED program for the first two weeks. Since a growing number of the population has an intolerance to wheat, I want to completely detox the body from wheat for the first two weeks, before reintroducing it back into the program. However, once wheat is brought back into your diet, you must pay close attention to how your body reacts. If you suffer any adverse reactions like nausea, headaches, bloating, sinus drip, phlegm, gas, or weight gain, then odds are you are allergic or have an intolerance to wheat and possibly gluten products as well. Should this be the case, then you'll have to cut wheat/gluten containing products from your diet. Rice, buckwheat, and millet would be good choices for you. Oats, barley, rye, and spelt all contain gluten just like wheat. Oats don't actually contain gluten; however, they are manufactured with other gluten containing grains. Celiac's disease is a severe allergic reaction to wheat/gluten products and can cause numerous health problems. For those with Celiac's disease, foods containing gluten should be avoided completely. The grains I allow back into the program are: Ezekiel bread (sprouted wheat), brown rice and oats. This way you can notice how your body feels without having too many choices to confuse issues. If a problem arises you may substitute in millet bread for the Ezekiel. More grain/carb foods are added later on in the program.

Whole grains provide B vitamins, vitamin E, and several minerals. They are also a good source of fiber and protein. Grains are also considered the main-burning fuel and are a good source of complex carbohydrates, which are slower burning and provide more sustained energy than simple carbohydrates. Grains have been around for over ten thousand years and are the most commonly consumed foods on earth. Too much of a good thing though, can cause problems resulting in the body becoming intolerant to it. The rotation concept is very important because you want to give your body a break every once in awhile from foods you consume regularly, if you don't you can become intolerant to that food. Try to vary your food choices daily. Don't eat your favorite food choices all the time; instead broaden your horizons by trying new foods, to ensure that you don't become intolerant to the foods you favor most.

Dairy

Like grains, dairy is not allowed during the first few weeks of the FED program. It is not reintroduced until week five. I chose to completely rid the body of dairy before bringing it back into the program for the same reasons as wheat. If intolerance is going to occur, then you will have symptoms such as bloating, nausea, headaches, constipation or diarrhea, and excess mucus. If these symptoms occur, discontinue dairy products immediately. Nearly half of the world's population is lactose intolerant. There are two other milk proteins, which can cause sensitivities as well, lactalbumin and milk casein. Milk is probably the most common food allergen and can cause various symptoms such as, rashes, ear infections, eczema, and hyperactivity, especially in children. According to Elson Haas, M.D., the over consumption of dairy products can contribute to congestive problems and degenerative diseases later in life. It is my experience that dairy products should be used as if they were a condiment, very sparingly. Cheeses alone are eighty percent fat, (mainly saturated unhealthy fats), and are also high in cholesterol.

Milk alternatives are rapidly becoming popular to the health conscious. Goat's milk, soy milk, rice milk, and almond milk are the most common choices. One of my favorites is a combination of soy and rice. The dairy choices that will be allowed in week five are part-skim ricotta cheese, mozzarella cheese, goat cheese, low-fat cottage cheese, and unsweetened organic plain yogurt.

The greatest nutrient we obtain from dairy products is calcium. There are also B vitamins, vitamins A, D, and E, along with several other minerals. As far as I am concerned, the cons for dairy products far outweigh the pros. I personally feel that by cutting out dairy altogether, you would be doing your body a great health service, however, if you are going to consume dairy products make sure that they are organic. One of the dairy products I used to recommend was yogurt – that is until I discovered how unhealthy commercial yogurt was. As I mentioned earlier in the previous chapter, the most touted health benefits are the beneficial bacteria, or live cultures contained in yogurt, however, not enough is in one container of yogurt to promote probiotic health. Acidophilus and bifidis are usually the two strains of bacteria that are used. Nowhere on the carton does it tell us exactly how much bacteria we will consume by eating a container of yogurt. Commercial brands of yogurt are also filled with sugar, usually in the form of high fructose corn syrup, or (equally as bad) plain ole sugar. There are a whopping 42 grams of sugar in one 8 oz. container, not to mention the food-coloring agents and the preservatives. I only recommend eating yogurt if it is organic and plain with no added sugar. You can always sweeten it yourself with fruit, all-fruit preserves, or Stevia.

Eggs

Eggs are definitely a large part of the FED program. And before I go any further, I want to clear up a tremendous misconception about eggs and cholesterol. Research shows that when eggs are consumed on a regular basis by themselves, and are not associated with a high-saturated fat diet, they will not raise serum cholesterol. I would only use caution for someone with a severe cholesterol problem or cardiovascular disease. The remedy for these people would be to eat only the egg white, which is where over half the protein is. The cholesterol is contained within the yolk. Eggs are a good source of vitamin A, all the B vitamins, D, E, and several minerals including, calcium and phosphorus for bone health. I encourage you to try eggs a number of different ways. Hard-boiled eggs are probably the easiest to prepare, and can be stored for use during the week. Omelets are delicious when made with any of these vegetables: mushrooms, fresh spinach, steamed broccoli, onions, garlic, all peppers, or tomatoes. They can be prepared, poached or soft boiled, over-easy, sunny-side-up, or plain ole scrambled, however, don't cook eggs over a high heat as this causes oxidation. Some people have an allergic reaction to eggs. If you get queasy or nauseous immediately after having eggs, you are probably one of these people. If this is the case, you may substitute a half ounce (twelve nuts) of almonds, or walnuts for a snack where a hard-boiled egg is suggested; and for breakfast you may sub in two ounces of lean protein, plus one teaspoon of flaxseed oil. These two suggestions will help keep you within the nutritional parameters of the FED program.

Animal Protein

This is the portion of the program where we lose the vegetarians. I am what you call a piscopolarian, and as I mentioned before, these are people who are primarily vegetarian, but will also consume fish and poultry. I tried being a strict vegetarian and had adverse reactions to the diet. My greatest concern was that I gained weight from all the grains and legumes that I had to eat, to meet my protein requirement. I am better off personally, as a piscopolarian. Protein requirements for the FED program are twenty to twenty-two percent of the program. The choices for animal protein are: lean beef, chicken, turkey, deep sea fish and canned chunk light tuna or sardines (low-sodium). No shellfish like clams, oysters, scallops, and mussels, or crustaceans such as, lobster, crab, or shrimp are allowed on the program because they are referred to as the scavengers of the sea, therefore, are high in contaminants like cadmium, mercury, and a whole slue of other toxins. Swordfish, king mackerel, grouper, and shark are also to be avoided due to the high level of mercury. Pork is to be avoided because of the associated health hazards such as, the prevalence of bacteria and parasites in pork. Cured pork products contain high-sodium and nitrates, which when digested become highly carcinogenic. Luncheon meats are also known for nitrites, high-sodium, unhealthy fats and a plethora of additives, coloring agents, and preservatives; therefore, it is best to avoid all of these unhealthy food choices.

Cooking techniques for meat would include, pan-frying or searing, baking, grilling, or broiling. The same goes for poultry and fish. Whenever you grill foods make sure that you do not burn them, because charred foods are carcinogenic. I usually brush a little olive oil on the food, whether it's meat or vegetable, apply spices liberally and then watch it carefully on the grill, turning it several times to prevent burning. This will ensure even cooking.

We get a wide variety of nutrients from red meat. Iron is probably the most touted nutrient associated with red meat. It is a form of iron that is more usable by our body then any other form of iron. Other nutrients include: the B vitamins, zinc and selenium, and vitamins A, D, and E, and a few other minerals as well. Poultry, specifically chicken and turkey, provides us with the B vitamins, vitamin A, and several minerals. Turkey is a little higher in zinc, iron, and potassium. Fish, however, is going to be the nutrient hero in the protein category. It is a higher source of protein than meat or poultry, and contains EFAs (essential fatty acids), also referred to as vitamin F. There are two categories for EFAs. These categories are omega 3 and omega 6. Omega-3 EFAs include alpha-linolinec and eicosapentaenoic acid (EPA), and are found in abundance in deep water fish like, salmon and sardines. Docosahexaenoic acid (DHA) and EPA are both powerful EFAs that help to reduce cholesterol and protect us from cardiovascular disease. They are called essential, because they have to be supplied through diet. Fish is also lower in fat as compared to red meat. Good delicious choices for fish are, cod, snapper, halibut, salmon, tilapia, sardines, and canned chunk light tuna.

Fats

The fat portion of the FED program is approximately thirty percent of the diet. The fats that are allowed on this program are: a polyunsaturated oil called Flaxseed oil, and olive oil, which is monounsaturated oil. There is a wealth of medicinal properties in flaxseed including, lowering blood pressure, cholesterol and triglycerides, aids in the prevention of arthritis and cardiovascular disease, and is essential for proper brain function. It is also beneficial in the treatment of eczema and psoriasis. Olive oil on the other hand has the ability to lower cholesterol's LDL levels, while raising the good HDL levels and also shares some of the same health benefits of flaxseed. Both of these oils are very important factors for disease prevention. The rest of the fat will come from eggs, animal protein and fish. I also recommend evening primrose oil or black current oil, which are both good sources of gamma-linolenic acid (GLA), however, those that have a history of breast cancer should use the black current oil because of evening primrose oil's estrogenic qualities, such as promoting the production of estrogen. This is the reason why evening primrose is recommended for the symptoms of menopause, by helping to reduce hot flashes. GLA supports the liver, thus promoting weight loss.

The use of olive oil spray, for cooking, is permitted because polyunsaturated oils, such as flaxseed, are heat sensitive, therefore, you cannot cook with them. Use olive oil and olive oil spray for cooking to avoid the creation of harmful fats. Flaxseed oil must be refrigerated. Other fats will be added back in after the seventh week of the program.

Beverages, Including Alcohol

The most important beverage for the FED program is water. The daily requirement is 8 eight-ounce glasses. Upon waking you will consume 8 oz. of warm water with lemon or lime. This beverage is what I call "the neutralizer." Acid/Alkaline balance is something I take very seriously. I see a lot of clients who are ill in my practice and when I test them for acid/alkaline balance, the majority of them are borderline acidosis, meaning their body is too acidic. Cancer thrives in an acidic atmosphere, so it is of vital importance to learn how to keep your body hovering around a healthy PH of 7.4, which is slightly alkaline. PH refers to the "potential of hydrogen," and is measured on a scale that ranges from one to fourteen. One is the overly acidic (acidosis) end of the spectrum, whereas fourteen is the very alkaline end, with seven being neutral. Water is neutral and citrus such as, lemon or lime is alkaline making this combination a great neutralizer, especially at the beginning and at the end of the day.

You will also be drinking unsweetened cranberry juice mixed with water as part of your water intake. Cranberry is important from a disease prevention and weight loss point of view. The health benefits are numerous. Cranberry has diuretic properties for detoxification, protects us from bacterial and viral infections of the urinary tract and the bladder, prevents cancer by preventing cellular damage with the aid of ellagic acid, has antifungal properties that strengthen the immune system, and is an excellent source of vitamin C and fiber. I will be reiterating these powerful properties, and those of all the foods and beverages, throughout the eight-week program. I want you to truly understand that "you are what you eat."

Other beverages allowed on the program are the limited use of unsweetened soy milk, and one cup of decaf coffee, but only if absolutely necessary. Caffeine is NOT allowed on the FED program. This includes: coffee, tea, colas, diet colas, chocolate, and caffeine stimulants (vivarin). Caffeine causes depletion of vital nutrients like B vitamins, calcium, magnesium, and iron, not to mention the fact that caffeine consumption will suppress immune function and will also increase your risk for kidney stones, gastrointestinal disorders, cardiovascular disease, fibrocystic breast disease, cancer, and will also hinder weight loss efforts because caffeine over-stresses the liver. Herbal tea and decaffeinated green tea is allowed during the program after week three, as well as pure orange juice in week four.

Alcohol is not good for anyone especially, liquor. It affects the central nervous system working as a sedative or depressant, which is why it makes people loosen up, after consuming only a couple of drinks. This happens from alcohol's sedation of the usual inhibitory mechanisms. It causes us to make poor judgments and say and do things that we, under normal circumstances, wouldn't dream of. It is unfortunate that some of us don't seem to have a cut off switch, when it comes to consuming alcohol, which leads to overuse and eventually alcoholism – a devastating disease. The FED program, however, allows limited use of some alcohol, beer and wine to be specific. FED recommends using lower alcohol wines, such as Reisling, Moscato, and light-wine blends. Check alcohol percentages on individual bottles. I also highly recommend organic wines because of the massive over-spraying of pesticides in vineyards. Light beers, or low-carb choices are preferred for beer. There are no other beverages allowed on the FED program.

Sugar

The only allowable sugars on the FED program are Stevia and Splenda. As I've stated before, this program is geared to detoxify your body from various toxins and chemicals, as well as sugar. Sugar feeds and breeds disease. There are no exceptions and I ask you to abstain from all sugar, other then those listed, for the duration of the program. This means no cake, cookies, ice cream, desserts of any kind, candy, gum, cough drops (use natural unsweetened drops, if needed), power bars, condiments (except for those listed in the program), juices, jams, and waters or beverages sweetened with aspartame. As I mentioned before, Aspartame, which consists of the combination of two amino acids aspartate, and phenylalanine, are referred to as exitotoxins, which kill brain neurons when taken in excess. No artificial sweeteners of any kind are allowed. Stevia and Splenda are considered natural sweeteners. High fructose corn syrup is also NOT allowed on this program. HFCS is stored as fat in the body because the body doesn't recognize it as a sugar to be burned as fuel. Make sure you read labels and know exactly what you are consuming.

Spices

NO salt is allowed during the first two weeks of the FED program. This was a very difficult task for me to cut salt from my diet. I am truly a salt-a-holic. I soon discovered that there were actually a few foods that I no longer liked, since I couldn't add salt to them; however, I do make a few exceptions for foods like eggs and meat. Table salt contains chemical additives and is processed at twelve hundred degrees, which drastically changes its chemical structure, therefore it should be avoided. Natural unprocessed sea salt is the only allowable salt on the program, but only when absolutely needed after the first two weeks. I found it really helped me to break my habit, when I stopped bringing the saltshaker to the table. In the place of salt I strongly encourage you to add liberal amounts of spices. There are certain warming spices that are called thermogenic, meaning that they raise the body's temperature thus raise metabolism. These spices include cayenne, ginger, turmeric, cumin, cinnamon, and mustard. A Cajun blend will also achieve this effect. Cinnamon is a good spice to add to fruit. It helps regulate blood sugar levels. Garlic is added to just about every meal I cook. Garlic has wonderful medicinal properties and is touted as one of the most treasured foods on earth. Garlic helps to lower blood pressure, thins the blood, which reduces the risk of clotting, lowers serum cholesterol levels, supports the immune system, and is natures most prized antibiotic. It is also antifungal, antibacterial, antiviral, and is good for the heart, colon, arthritis, and circulation. I personally use it to help keep my allergies in check, especially, during hay fever season. Other herbs and spices such as, basil, oregano, thyme, coriander, tarragon, chives, and bay leaf also have great medicinal properties. Be adventurous and spice it up!

This covers all the food groups you will be consuming during the FED program. You will be given further information on the particulars of these food groups in the next chapter.

Testimonial

Grant

My name is Grant and I am a medical technician. I started the FED program in early February at my place of business. I was hopeful that by changing the way I was eating, I could learn to correct my GERD (acid reflux) problem. Two days on the program I stopped taking my Axid (acid blocker) and haven't had an episode of heartburn/acid, since. That was a month and a half ago. I didn't have a lot of weight to lose, but I went from a size thirty-eight waist, to a size thirty-four waist in three weeks on the program. My cholesterol levels have also dropped quite a bit. I feel great and am grateful to my co-workers for talking me into joining the FED program (but don't tell them that). Thanks a lot FED!

Chapter Five

Segments One-Three, The Beginning Of Change

Now that you have learned about foods and supplements you will be consuming, you are ready to begin the FED program. The first two weeks are the most crucial for the detoxification process. I strongly urge you to slowly wean yourself off caffeine the week prior to beginning this program. After giving up caffeine two years ago, I personally found that cutting your caffeine in half (half caffeinated to half decaf) is a good start to coming off caffeine. Slowly begin adding in more decaf until you have completely omitted caffeine. This goes for tea, cola, and diet cola, as well.

During the first few days of week one you may experience fatigue or a headache. These symptoms are part of the detoxification process. I have had some of my clients experience these symptoms and some that didn't. This is the body's natural reaction to the elimination of caffeine, sugar, sodium, wheat, dairy, additives, preservatives, and coloring agents. These symptoms are temporary and you shouldn't be concerned. It is simply your body rejoicing to this wonderful change in diet. These symptoms improve after a day or two and somewhere around day 14 you will experience a wonderful increase in energy.

The second week on the program is when it happened for me. Prior to beginning the program, I thought I had chronic fatigue syndrome. Every day at around two o'clock in the afternoon, I would get so sleepy that I felt I needed to nap. I remember sitting at my desk one day and suddenly the realization dawned on me, it was after two o'clock and didn't feel tired; as a matter of fact I felt great. The FED program has become a way of life for me. When I started the program I had fifteen pounds to lose. Slowly over the last two years I allowed my weight to creep back up to where I started feeling the effects of carrying around fifteen pounds of excess baggage. I dropped the weight pretty quickly on the FED program. The first fourteen days I lost eight and a half pounds. By week four I was down eleven pounds and lost the next four pounds by the end of the eight weeks. I have not only lost the weight but consequently I lost six inches of fat from all over my body, and came back down to a size 6. This is a story that you too will experience over the next few weeks. You can expect a reduction in clothing size after just a few weeks on the program.

In case you are wondering when I am going to talk about the exercise requirements for the FED program, the time is now. Exercising is definitely encouraged during the entire program and on through maintenance, however, it is limited to thirty minutes per day, three times per week for the first three weeks and then you can increase up to five times weekly. The reason is because of what we discussed in chapter one pertaining to your basal metabolic rate (BMR). It is imperative that you don't burn more fuel than you are taking in. This will greatly upset your metabolism and we want to avoid that.

The best time to exercise is first thing in the morning, however, some people find their schedules don't allow for an added morning routine, so exercising whenever you can fit it in would be just fine. Exercise doesn't have to be a chore. I joined Curves for Women, and go two to three times weekly. On the days that I am not at curves, I enjoy a morning walk with my dog, Jack. Walking gives me time to quiet the mind, and just enjoy the beauty around me. Dancing and biking are also some of my favorite forms of exercise. One of my clients has five young children and is running around constantly after them and if she's not doing that, then she's busy cleaning the house. I told her that was plenty of exercise for her and then some, although, I did recommended yoga two to three times weekly, as well as asked her to incorporate some form of meditation into her busy life. It is vital to take time for ourselves. Those of us that are constant care givers to others and neglect ourselves are the ones that get sick. I can't tell you how many cancer clients have told me that they are the ones that everyone turns to for help, and that they never have the time to take care of themselves. If you fall into this category, now is the time to change your ways. You have made the decision to take on the FED program to regain your health, so make sure you take the time to give it your all. Do this for your whole body. The mind goes hand in hand with the body and spirit. I will discuss this more in depth later on in the book.

Now that you are ready, let's begin the FED program. Over the next several pages you will find segments 1-3. Each segment is broken down into two-week intervals. Weeks one and two will be the same as far as structure goes, with a daily meal plan that will be referred to throughout the program. Weeks three and four begin the reintroduction of grain, and weeks five and six will introduce some dairy choices. It is very important that you adhere to the program to the best of your ability the first two weeks. This is when you will be detoxing, and setting your body up for the rest of the program. Remember to use organic foods as much as possible and to eat all your vegetables. Vegetables are a large part of your disease preventative foods, as well as your disease fighters. You will continue to use all recommended supplements throughout the program, unless otherwise stated. Make sure you read everything contained in each given week, especially the italicized print. Frozen fruits and vegetables are permitted when time is a factor. However, I prefer that you use fresh as much as possible.

I have personally found that GNC (General Nutrition Centers) carries just about all the supplements needed for the FED program. They even have the flaxseed oil and the unsweetened cranberry juice. You can also purchase these supplements from your local health food store. I have also listed a few mail-order companies for your convenience. You will find this information in the resource section of this book.

For your beverage consumption, I have found that it is a tremendous time saver to make a 48 oz. pitcher of the unsweetened cranberry juice (your daily amount). This will be your requirement for the first two weeks. This takes the pressure off of trying to keep track of how much you consumed, unless of course you decide to use the FED food diary.

I believe I have covered all aspects of the program up to this point. A question and answer section is included in chapter eight. I would also like to reiterate once more that we are all human and to err is human. If you jump ship just climb back on board and continue where you left off. Let's now begin week one.

To begin the program you will need to figure out you Basal Metabolic Rate (BMR). Meals are based on three options; if you have a basal metabolic rate (BMR) between 1200 and 1600, use 4 oz. of protein for meals, if it falls between 1600 and 2000, use 6 oz. of protein for meals. For those of you that have a higher BMR (between 2000 and 2400), use 8 oz. of protein per given meal; and add one extra egg to the breakfast meal. Vegetable allowances will also increase (see food plan for increase). This allows for the additional calories needed for BMR. Refer to chapter one to find out your BMR. (An important note here: remember to recheck your Basal Metabolic Rate as you lose weight since your BMR will change.)

I have included a weight reference chart for men and women on the following page. Pick a realistic goal weight. If you have a lot of weight to lose, I recommend that you pick a short-term goal first. For example: if you are 5'5 and weigh 180 pounds and are 50 years of age, your ideal weight range should fall between 117-155 pounds depending on your age and frame. Make your first goal 155 pounds, then you can begin to work your way down from there should you choose to. Keep in mind that the weight charts on the following pages are for reference only. How you feel at a certain weight and your overall health status is what really matters.

WEIGHT CHART

WOMEN-Weighed Clothed - Age 21-60

Small		Medium	Large
4'11	103-113	111-123	120-134
5'0	104-115	113-126	122-137
5'1	106-118	115-129	125-140
5'2	108-121	118-132	128-143
5'3	111-124	121-135	131-147
5'4	114-127	124-138	134-151
5'5	117-130	127-141	137-155
5'6	120-133	130-144	140-159
5'7	123-136	133-147	143-163
5'8	126-139	136-150	146-167
5'9	129-142	139-153	149-170
5'10	132-145	142-156	152-173
5'11	135-148	145-159	155-176

WEIGHT CHART

MEN-Weighed Clothed - Age 21-60

Small		Medium	Large
5'1	126-132	129-138	136-147
5'0	124-130	127-135	134-143
5'2	128-134	131-141	138-150
5'3	130-136	133-143	140-153
5'4	132-138	135-145	142-156
5'5	134-140	137-148	144-160
5'6	136-142	139-151	146-164
5'7	138-145	142-154	149-168
5'8	140-148	145-157	153-172
5'9	142-151	148-160	155-176
5'10	144-154	151-163	158-180
5'11	146-157	154-166	161-184
6'0	149-160	157-170	164-188
6'1	152-164	160-174	168-192
6'2	155-168	164-178	172-197
6'3	158-172	167-182	176-2

FAT ELIMINATION AND DETOX PROGRAM
Segment 1/ Weeks 1 & 2

Supplements

*Good quality multi-vitamin/mineral.

*Flaxseed Oil (EFA) - 1 tablespoon daily. (Protects against many diseases: cancer, cardiovascular, arthritis; supports all body systems and lowers cholesterol and triglyceride levels.)

*Evening Primrose or Black Currant Oil (GLA) - as directed daily. (Similar properties as flaxseed oil + aiding in weight loss and is beneficial to the liver.) Refer to chapter three to determine which GLA you should take.

*Lecithin Granules - 1 tablespoon daily. (Important fats called phospholipids for cellular health, energy and maintenance of cholesterol levels, as well as a good source of phosphatidylcholine for brain function and fat metabolism.)

*For those individuals with digestive difficulties, I also recommend probiotics (Nature's Way Primadophilis) and a good digestive enzyme to be taken with meals (Digest Gold by Enzymedica). These will aid in the digestion and elimination process.

Program Foods and Beverages For First Segment:

Beverages

*8 oz. warm water with fresh lemon juice in a.m. and p.m. (Nutrient rich fruit high in vitamins B, C, E, and several minerals. Terpenes help regulate cholesterol and enzymes that may promote tumor growth. Also balances acid/alkaline levels and aids in elimination for detoxification.)

*2 oz. unsweetened cranberry juice with 6 oz. clean filtered water (not cold) 6 times daily. (This is a diuretic, good source of ellagic acid for the prevention of cellular damage that can lead to cancer, and for prevention of cystitis and bladder infections by keeping bacteria from attaching to the cells that line the bladder and urinary tract. Cranberries have antifungal and antiviral properties that strengthen the immune system. Good source of vitamin C and fiber.)

*1 cup decaf coffee in the a.m. (if necessary), and absolutely no caffeine. (Caffeine depletes the body of vital nutrients especially the B vitamins calcium, magnesium and iron and also puts you at risk for kidney stones, gastrointestinal problems, cardiac problems, and FBD (fibrocystic breast disease). Most of all, caffeine will hinder weight loss due to over-stressing the liver.)

*Never drink beverages with meal, drink at the end of meals or prior to. This is to avoid diluting digestive juices and enzymes.

Vegetables: (Organic if possible)

8-10 cups (1200-1600 BMR), 10-12 cups (1600-2000 BMR), and 12-14 cups (2000-2400 BMR).

(Include celery for its diuretic and laxative properties. Good insoluble fiber source).

Cancer fighting; green leafy vegetables, cruciferous vegetables (broccoli, cauliflower, cabbage, bok choy, etc.), onions, garlic (include this ancient healing food to lower blood pressure, the risk for heart disease and cancer. Garlic also has immune-building properties; is anti-microbial and is known as nature's antibiotic), mushrooms and carrots. Avoid potatoes (all), corn, winter squash, peas, soybeans (edamame), and pumpkin for the first 2 weeks.

Fruits (Organic if possible)

3 choices daily (all BMR groups)

Portion examples are as follows:
1 cup berries, 5 dried apricots, 2 medium pieces of fruit or 1 large fruit = 1 serving

Choose high-fiber fruit; berries (good source for ellagic acid to prevent cellular damage that can lead to cancer, blueberries, cranberries and strawberries (organic only) are the best choices), apples (good source of soluble and insoluble fiber, health benefits include sugar stabilizer, and cholesterol reducer), apricots (high in beta carotene for lowering cholesterol and blood pressure, macular degeneration, cataracts, and improves night vision), kiwi, (high source for vitamin C), and cherries (good when craving sugar and a good source of fiber).

NOTE: Apples, all berries, cherries, lemon, grapefruit, apricots, and peaches are the preferred fruit choices for this segment. High glycemic fruits are to be avoided, such as bananas, grapes, raisins, figs, pineapple, watermelon, etc.

Grains

None during this segment.

Dairy

None during this segment.

Eggs

1-2 daily (all BMR groups, except those at 2000-2400 add 1 additional egg daily).

If eggs are a problem, then you may substitute 2 oz. of lean protein: chicken, turkey or fish + 1 teaspoon of flaxseed oil (this is in addition to the 2 tablespoons of flaxseed oil on the program), although I prefer you do the eggs.

Chicken eggs, preferably organic, free roaming (Good source of protein, lutein, and choline, Vitamins A, D, E, and B, lecithin, zinc, and calcium).

Note: Eggs do not contribute to cholesterol levels if they are not associated with a high saturated fat diet.

Animal Protein Sources

8-16 oz. daily (depending on BMR)

Lean beef (Maverick Ranch free roam), Poultry (Springer Mountain Farms free roam), Fish (deep ocean) Publix frozen varieties: cod, snapper, Coho salmon (a rich source of EFA's), haddock, halibut, orange roughy, and mahi. You can use low-sodium canned chunk light tuna or sardines.

Fats

One tablespoon flaxseed oil and 1 tablespoon of olive oil daily. You may use olive oil spray for cooking.

NOTE: Never cook with flaxseed oil. Polyunsaturated oils are easily damaged by heat and light and must be refrigerated.

Alcohol

None (For the first two weeks).

Sugar

Stevia, Splenda (absolutely NO sugar).

Spices (Organic if possible).

NO salt! Use these beneficial herbs instead: Coriander, **cayenne, ginger, cinnamon,** garlic, onion, **turmeric,** curry, celery seed, **cumin,** fennel, **mustard,** basil, and oregano. Many of these (bold print) are called thermogenic, meaning they raise the body temperature; thus your metabolism. They are all powerful disease fighters and have many medicinal properties. (Sea salt may be used sparingly, for eggs and meats only if necessary.)

Considerations

All of the above food sources are loaded with vital nutrients that are required daily for the body to function properly however; the multivitamin is our added insurance to ensure we are getting everything we need.

Exercising is encouraged for the elimination process of toxins through the lymphatic system and to raise your metabolism, however, during the first two weeks exercise for no longer than thirty minutes with five minutes of stretching three times per week. It is imperative NOT to burn more energy (calories) than the body will allow because the body will start hoarding calories. Walking is the preferred form of exercise.

Time saving tips: Steam or sauté veggies ahead of time and refrigerate. Try to consume plenty of raw veggies as well, for enzyme and fiber retaining properties. You can also prepare chicken and other protein choices in advance to save time. For example: a cooked whole turkey will last all week in the refrigerator and will be ready to eat as needed. I also boil eggs on the weekend for the following week.

NOTE: If you consume lean protein for breakfast, then have two hardboiled eggs for lunch and vice versa. Make sure you rotate your breakfast choices.

DAILY MENU- (Increase BMR Food choices accordingly as per individual food category)

Upon Waking: 8 oz. warm water with ½ squeezed lemon (for alkalizing).

Breakfast

(Alternate choices daily)

2 egg omelet with spinach and mushrooms (or any veggies) made with olive oil spray. (Or 2 eggs any style). Celery sticks. 8 oz. cranberry water.

OR

2 oz. lean protein like turkey, beef, chicken, or fish, + 1 teaspoon of flaxseed oil. Sliced tomatoes with steamed asparagus. 8 oz. cranberry water.

OR

Fruit smoothie made with two scoops of hemp protein powder or Nature's Plus Source of Life Energy Shake powder + 1 cup water, 1 cup of fruit, and ½-1 packet of Stevia/Splenda OR you may use 1 cup of unsweetened Westsoy or Silk soy milk, + 1 cup of fruit (berries, cherries or peaches) and Stevia/Splenda. If fruit is frozen, no ice is needed, if fresh, add 4-6 ice cubes. 8 oz. cranberry water.

10 a.m. - 1 serving of fruit or a hard-boiled egg.

NOTE: If you had a smoothie earlier then choose an egg for this snack.

Lunch

4-8 oz. lean protein, + unlimited vegetables.
If consuming a salad, use 1 T. flaxseed oil, 1 T. apple cider vinegar, 1 T. water, lemon juice, crushed garlic,

spices, and sweetener if needed.

OR

Stir-fry: use a small amount of olive oil spray with a little water to sauté vegetables. Then drizzle with 1 tablespoon of flaxseed oil over top. 8 oz. cranberry water.

Alternate salad dressing recipe:

Honey Mustard (minus the honey)

1T. prepared mustard (wheat-free)
1T. apple cider vinegar
1T. flaxseed oil
½ T. water
½ packet Stevia/Splenda
Shake vigorously.

NOTE: Plan ahead and make extra. When dining out bring a small single serving size container for your dressing, instead of ordering the dressing on the menu.

2 p.m. - 16 oz. cranberry water.

4 p.m. - Cranberry waterw/lemon.

Dinner

4-8 oz. lean protein (if you had meat for lunch, have fish for dinner), + stir-fry, steamed, or sautéed vegetables and a salad. 8 oz. cranberry water w/ lemon (if desired).

NOTE: Be adventurous and try new vegetables. Make sure you only use 2 tablespoons of oil daily. Whether it's drizzled or used in dressing, it counts!

8 p.m. - 1 cup of peaches, OR, ¾ cup blueberries
OR, 5 dried apricots. (a good fiber source)

Before Bed - 8 oz. warm lemon water.

Now repeat week one for the second week in segment one.

FED FOOD DIARY

SUPPLEMENTS- Flax __ GLA __ Multi __ __ Lecithin __

BREAKFAST-

LUNCH-

DINNER-

SNACKS-

(Check off food categories)

FRUIT - __ __ __

EGGS - __ __ __

PROTEIN - (per 2 oz.) __ __ __ __ __ __ __ __

WATER/JUICE - __ __ __ __ __ __ __ __

CARBS/GRAINS - __ __

DAIRY - __ __

VEGETABLES - __ __ __ __ __ __ __ __ __ __ __ __ __ __

FAT - (per tablespoon) - __ __

FED GROCERY SHOPPING LIST- SEGMENT 1

Supplements

Flax seed oil,
Evening Primrose oil or Black Current oil
Multivitamin/mineral
Lecithin
Unsweetened Cranberry juice
Protein powder (if not using soy milk as base)

Produce (I strongly Recommend Organic Produce)

(Choose from the following lists)
Broccoli
Cauliflower
Green beans
Onions
Garlic
Tomatoes
Romaine or other dark green lettuce (not iceberg)
Cucumbers
Sprouts (clover, alfalfa, sunflower, or broccoli)
Zucchini
Summer squash
Carrots
Bok Choy
Cabbage
Apples
Cherries

Blueberries/ Black or Raspberries
Strawberries
Peaches

Nectarines
Plums
Pears
Dried prunes or apricots
Kiwi
Lemon
Lime

Animal Protein/Eggs (free-range)

Eggs
Springer Mountain Farms Chicken
Maverick Ranch Beef
Deep sea frozen or fresh fish (see program for choices)

Fats

Flax seed oil (also listed in supplements)
Olive oil
Olive oil cooking spray

Sugar

Stevia
Splenda

Miscellaneous

Unsweetened soy milk, regular, vanilla, and chocolate

FAT ELIMINATION AND DETOX PROGRAM
Segment 2/Week 3

Supplements

Same as before.

Beverages

*8 oz. warm water with ½ squeezed lemon in a.m. and p.m.

*2 oz. unsweetened cranberry juice with 6 oz. clean filtered water 2 times daily.

*4-8 oz. glasses of clean filtered water daily. Can include 1 cup of decaffeinated tea (green or herbal preferred).

*1 cup of decaffeinated coffee in the a.m. (if necessary) does not count toward water intake.

Vegetables

8-10 cups/10-12 cups/12-14 cups daily (depending on BMR)

Same as before but you may add in once daily ½ cup peas, edamame (soybeans are a rich source of phytoestrogens, a weaker version of the hormone estrogen we produce naturally, that helps to keep raging estrogen in check; normalizing levels), ½ ear of corn, or a small yam or ½ small sweet potato (excellent source of fiber and beta-carotene).

Note: Work these new vegetable choices in as part of your vegetable allowances not in addition to. Also note that yams are allowed first over sweet potatoes, because of the glycemic index and because sweet potatoes have nearly double the amount of calories.

Fruits

Same as before.

Grains

1 choice daily.

Add in ½ cup brown rice, not instant, (rice bran contains the compound orysanol, which reduces the production of cholesterol) or oatmeal or oat bran, ½ cup (dry before cooking) can use instant if necessary, 1 ½ packets - no sodium only! Oats have powerful compounds called saponins, which bind to and eliminate cholesterol and cholesterol-containing bile), or 1 slice of Ezekiel low-sodium bread daily. (Good source of protein and fiber.)

Note: If you have one of the added vegetables for this segment, then do not combine them at the same meal as your grain choice, 1 vegetable starch and 1 grain choice at separate meals daily.

Also pay attention to how your body feels after consuming wheat or gluten products (Ezekiel bread or oats). Bloating, gas, diarrhea, constipation, nausea, dermatitis, or sluggishness may indicate intolerance or Celiacs's disease. If any of these symptoms occur, eliminate these food choices immediately. If this is the case, then sub in 1 slice millet bread and quinoa for oats.

Nuts

½ oz. daily (to be substituted for egg snack).

½ oz. almonds (12 whole almonds - helps prevent heart disease and lowers cholesterol; also a good source of vitamin E, copper, magnesium, good fats and protein) or, walnuts (walnuts - good source of EFA linoleic and alpha-linoeic acids, they also contain a powerful antioxidant called ellagic acid that is known to fight cancer cells; are chock full of selenium, zinc, vitamin E and iron).

NOTE: Remember to have nuts in place of hard boiled egg snack.

Peanuts are actually legumes and also referred to as a pea – hence the name peanut, and are also a good source of protein, good fat, B vitamins and several minerals. Stored peanuts, however, are known to have molds, specifically molds containing aflatoxin, which is carcinogenic. I recommend avoiding peanuts and never consuming fresh ground peanut butter, because of these molds.

Dairy

None added this segment.

Eggs

1-3 daily. (depending on BMR)

Animal Protein Sources

Same as before.

Fats

2 tablespoons daily.

1 tablespoon flaxseed oil and 1 tablespoon of olive oil daily.

Alcohol

1 - 4 oz. glass of red wine (organic preferred- red wine contains quercetin and resveratrol, powerful flavonoids, that have been proven to have even more heart protective effects than Vitamin E, also keeps dangerous LDL cholesterol from sustaining free radical damage while raising good HDL levels for overall heart disease prevention) in lieu of one fruit serving, 2-3

times weekly,

OR

1 - Low carb or light beer may be substituted for added carb/starch 2-3 times weekly.

Sugar

Same as before.

Spices

Same as before.

Considerations

Breakfast can now have 3 meal choices: 2 eggs (as listed on previous week list) with 1 slice of Ezekiel toast with drizzled flaxseed oil on it OR, 1½ packets or ½ cup (dry before cooked) oatmeal or oat bran (higher fiber content) sweetened with Stevia or Splenda + 2 tablespoons of unsweetened soy milk + ½ cup of unsweetened applesauce with cinnamon (to be eaten after the grain to level out blood sugar, counts as 1/2 fruit serving). These are the choices to alternate with the breakfast smoothie every other day.

Remember: Spend your new carb choices wisely.

FAT ELIMINATION AND DETOX PROGRAM
Segment 2/Week 4

Supplements

Same as before.

Beverages

*8 oz. warm water with ½ squeezed lemon in a.m. and p.m.

*2 oz. unsweetened cranberry juice with 6 oz. clean filtered water 2 times daily.

*4-8 oz. glasses of clean filtered water daily. You can include 1 cup of decaffeinated tea (green or herbal preferred).

*1 cup of decaffeinated coffee in the a.m. (if necessary) does not count toward water intake.

Vegetables

8-10 cups/10-12 cups/12-14 cups daily (depending on BMR)

Same as before but you may add in once daily ½ cup peas, edamame (soybeans are a rich source of phytoestrogens, a weaker version of the hormone estrogen we produce naturally, that helps to keep raging estrogen in check; normalizing levels), ½ ear of corn (high glycemic; use sparingly), ½ cup winter squash, OR a small yam or ½ small sweet potato (excellent source of fiber and beta-carotene, but higher glycemic factor only 2-3 times weekly), ½ cup of black or pinto beans (these high protein and high fiber, disease-fighting legumes are great tossed in salads in place of chicken or fish, or as a condiment to an egg breakfast. Do not consume with any other protein sources; impedes digestion. Benefits are numerous: they lower cholesterol, protect against cancer and heart disease and help stabilize blood sugar levels.)

Note: Work these new vegetable choices in as part of your vegetable allowances not in addition to. Also note that yams are allowed first over sweet potatoes because a sweet potato is higher on the glycemic chart and is almost double the calories of a yam.

Fruits

3 servings daily. Same choices as before + you may add in:

½ banana, small bunch of grapes, or 4 oz. orange juice 2-3 times weekly as 1 serving of fruit, (high glycemic fruit, use sparingly).

Grains

2 choices daily (1 choice per day; don't double up on the same carb.)

Add in ½ cup brown rice,or ½ cup oatmeal or oatbran (dry before cooking) can use instant if necessary, use 1½ packets - no sodium only; oats have powerful compounds called saponins, which bind to and eliminate cholesterol and cholesterol-containing bile) or 1 slice of Ezekiel low-sodium bread daily or comparable sprouted grain bread. (Good source of protein and fiber.)

(Note: if you have one of the added vegetables for this segment, then do not combine them at the same meal as your grain choice – 1 vegetable/ starch and 1 grain/starch at separate meals daily.) Also keep your meat/fish protein separate from grain carbs; they don't combine well together.

Also pay attention to how your body feels after consuming wheat or gluten products (Ezekiel bread or oats). Bloating, gas, constipation, or sluggishness may indicate intolerance or possibly Celiacs's disease. If this is the case then substitute 1 slice millet bread for the Ezekiel and quinoa for the oats.

Dairy

None added this segment.

Eggs

1-3 daily.

Nuts

½ *oz. daily* (to be substituted for egg snack)

½ oz. almonds (12 whole almonds- helps prevent heart disease and lowers cholesterol; also a good source of vitamin E, copper, magnesium, good fats and protein) or walnuts (walnuts- good source of EFA linoleic and alpha-linoeic acids, they also contain a powerful antioxidant called ellagic acid that's known to fight cancer cells; are chock full of selenium, zinc, vitamin E and iron).

Note: Remember to have nuts in place of hard boiled egg snack.

Animal Protein Sources

Same as before.

Fats

2 tablespoons daily.

1 tablespoon flaxseed oil and 1 tablespoon of olive oil daily.

Alcohol

Same as before.

OR

1- Low carb or light beer may substitute added carb/starch 2-3 times weekly.

Sugar

Same as before.

Spices

Same as before.

Considerations

Breakfast can now have 3 meal choices: 2 eggs (as listed on previous week list) with 1 slice of Ezekiel toast with drizzled flaxseed oil on it or, 1½ packets or ½ cup (dry before cooked) oatmeal or oat bran (higher fiber content) sweetened with Stevia or Splenda + 2 tablespoons of unsweetened soy milk + ½ cup of unsweetened applesauce with cinnamon (to be eaten after the grain to level out blood sugar, counts as 1/2 fruit serving). These are the choices to alternate with the breakfast smoothie every other day.

Remember: Spend your new carb choices wisely.

Exercise

Now is the time to increase your exercise to compensate for the additional calories added in this segment. Exercising three to five times weekly is highly encouraged, up to thirty minutes each day. Curves for Women is a great way to firm up and lose inches and walking is always a good choice. Spread workouts out over the week – DO NOT exercise three days in a row and then do nothing else for the rest of the week. It is important to spread them out.

FAT ELIMINATION AND DETOX PROGRAM
Segment 3/Week 5

Supplements

Same as before.

Digestive Enzymes – Digest Gold by Enzymedica as directed. (I recommend these, especially, in this segment with the reintroduction of dairy. Dairy is difficult for many people to digest, therefore, digestive enzymes will aid in the digestion process.)

Beverages

*8 oz. warm water with ½ squeezed lemon in a.m. and p.m.

*2 oz. unsweetened cranberry juice with 6 oz. clean filtered water 2 times daily.

*4-8 oz. glasses of clean filtered water daily. Can include 1 cup of decaffeinated tea (green or herbal preferred.)

*1 cup of decaffeinated coffee in the a.m. (if necessary) does not count toward water intake.

Vegetables

8-10 cups/10-12 cups/12-14 cups daily (depending on BMR)

Same as before but you may add in once daily ½ cup peas, edamame (soybeans are a rich source of phytoestrogens, a weaker version of the hormone estrogen we produce naturally, which helps to keep raging estrogen in check; normalizing levels), ½ ear of corn (high glycemic; use sparingly), ½ cup winter squash, OR a small yam or ½ small sweet potato (excellent source of fiber and beta-carotene, but higher glycemic factor only 2-3 times weekly), ½ cup of black or pinto beans (these high protein and high fiber, disease-fighting legumes are great tossed in salads in place of chicken or fish, or as a condiment to an egg breakfast. Do not consume with any other protein sources; impedes digestion. Benefits are numerous: lowers cholesterol, protects against cancer and heart disease and helps stabilize blood sugar levels.)

Note: Work these new vegetable choices in as part of your vegetable allowances not in addition to. Also note that yams are allowed first over sweet potatoes because of the glycemic index and because sweet potatoes have nearly double the amount of calories.

Fruits

3 servings daily. Same as before + you may add in:

½ banana, small bunch of grapes or 4 oz. orange juice 2-3 times weekly as 1 serving of fruit. (high-glycemic fruit, use sparingly).

Grains

Twice daily.

Add in ½ cup brown rice, OR ½ cup dry (before cooking) oatmeal, or oat bran (higher fiber), 1½ packets - instant no sodium only (oats have powerful compounds called saponins, which bind to and eliminate cholesterol and cholesterol-containing bile) or 1 slice of Ezekiel low-sodium bread daily. (Good source of protein and fiber.)

NOTE: If you have one of the added vegetables for this segment then do not combine them at the same meal as your grain choice - 1 vegetable starch and 1 grain choice at separate meals daily.) Also keep your meat/fish protein choices separate from grain/carbs; they don't combine well. Also note how your body feels. Determine if the second added carb is causing any health problems. If so, then decrease back to only one choice daily as long as you can tolerate it.

Dairy

1 choice daily. (organic preferred to eliminate growth-promoters/ hormones/antibiotics).

¼ cup part-skim ricotta cheese, 1 oz. part-skim mozzarella cheese, 1 oz. goat cheese or ¼ cup crumbled, 1 small cup (1/2 cup) organic unsweetened yogurt (may sweeten with Stevia/Splenda), OR, ½ cup low-fat low-sodium cottage cheese (lower in calories and fat than most cheeses and a good source of protein).

Note: Most cheeses have high fat content, mainly saturated, some as much as eighty percent fat, and are high in cholesterol and sodium, therefore are not considered a healthy disease preventative food choice. Be sure to read labels, know exactly what you're eating! Caution, if constipation, diarrhea, bloating, or excess phlegm occurs, eliminate dairy. You may be allergic or lactose intolerant.

Eggs

1 daily (unless dairy is a problem, then follow 1-3 eggs daily).

(This adjustment is needed because of the reintroduction of dairy, which is high in fat, but also a good protein source).

Nuts

1/2 oz. daily (to be substituted for egg snack)

½ oz. almonds (12 whole almonds–helps prevent heart disease and lowers cholesterol; also a good source of vitamin E, copper, magnesium, good fats and protein) or walnuts (walnuts- good source of EFA linoleic and alpha-linoeic acids, they also contain a powerful antioxidant called ellagic acid that's known to fight cancer cells; are chock full of selenium, zinc, vitamin E and iron).

NOTE: Remember to have nuts in place of hard boiled egg snack.

Animal Protein Sources

Same as before.

Fats

1 tablespoon + 2 teaspoons daily.

1 tablespoon flaxseed oil, and 2 teaspoons of olive oil daily.

(To compensate for the added dairy fat. If you choose NOT to add in second dairy choice, then allow 2 tablespoons daily, as before.)

Alcohol

Same as before.

OR

1- Low carb or light beer may substitute added carb/starch 2-3 times weekly.

Sugar

Same as before.

Spices

Same as before.

Considerations

Breakfast can now have 4 meal choices: 1 egg with 1 slice of Ezekiel toast with ¼ cup ricotta cheese spread on it- topped with 3 peach slices OR ¼ cup of fruit of choice, OR 1½ packets or ½ cup (dry before cooked) oatmeal or oat bran (higher fiber content) sweetened with Stevia or Splenda + 2 tablespoons of unsweetened soy milk + ½ cup of unsweetened applesauce with cinnamon (to be eaten after the grain to level out blood sugar levels; counts as 1/2 fruit serving) OR ½ cup of yogurt with 1 serving of fruit, and 1 slice of Ezekiel bread drizzled with flaxseed oil. These are the choices to alternate with the breakfast smoothie every other day.

Remember: Spend your new carb choices wisely, and consume fruit at the end of the meal to regulate blood sugar levels.

Continue exercising at least 30 minutes 3-5 times weekly.

FAT ELIMINATION AND DETOX PROGRAM
Segment 3/Week 6

Supplements

Same as before.

*Digestive Enzymes - Digest Gold by Enzymedica as directed. (I recommend these, especially, in this segment with the reintroduction of dairy. Dairy is difficult for many people to digest, therefore, digestive enzymes will aid in the digestion process.)

*Probiotics - I highly recommend incorporating probiotics (friendly bacteria) into your diet on a daily basis. Nature's Way Primadophilis is a good once-a-day probiotic. Health benefits include: assists in digestion, inhibits pathogenic organisms in the digestive tract, has antifungal properties, aids immune function, and enhances absorption of nutrients.

Beverages

*8 oz. warm water with ½ squeezed lemon in a.m. and p.m.

*2 oz. unsweetened cranberry juice with 6 oz. clean filtered water 2 times daily.

*4-8 oz. glasses of clean filtered water daily.
You can include 1 cup of decaffeinated tea (green or herbal preferred).

*1 cup of decaffeinated coffee in the a.m. (if necessary) does not count toward water intake.

Vegetables

8-10 cups/10-12 cups/12-14 cups daily, (depending on BMR).

Same as before but you may add in once daily ½ cup peas, edamame (soybeans are a rich source of phytoestrogens, a weaker version of the hormone estrogen we produce naturally that helps to keep raging estrogen in check; normalizing levels.), ½ ear of corn (high glycemic, use sparingly), ½ cup winter squash, or a small yam or ½ sweet potato (excellent source of fiber and beta-carotene), ½ cup of black or pinto beans (these high protein and high fiber, disease-fighting legumes are great tossed in salads in place of chicken or fish, or as a condiment to an egg breakfast. Do not consume with any other protein sources - impedes digestion. Benefits are numerous: lowers cholesterol, protects against cancer and heart disease and helps stabilize blood sugar levels.)

NOTE: Work these new vegetable choices in as part of your vegetable allowances not in addition to. Also note that yams are allowed over sweet potatoes because of the glycemic index and because sweet potatoes have nearly double the amount of calories.

Fruits

3 servings daily. Same as before + you may add in:

½ banana, small bunch of grapes, or 4 oz. orange juice, 2-3 times weekly as 1 serving of fruit. (all high-glycemic fruit, use sparingly).

Grains

Twice daily.

Add in ½ cup brown rice, OR ½ cup dry (before cooking) oatmeal or oat bran (higher in fiber) 1½ packets of instant oatmeal - no sodium only (oats have powerful compounds called saponins, which bind to and eliminate cholesterol and cholesterol-containing bile) OR 1 slice of Ezekiel low-sodium bread daily. (Good source of protein and fiber.)

NOTE: If you have one of the added vegetables for this segment, then do not combine them at the same meal as your grain choice – 1 vegetable starch and 1 grain choice at separate meals daily. Also don't combine grain/carb with meat/fish protein; they don't combine well for digestion. Also note how your body feels. Determine if the second added carb is causing any health problems. If so, then decrease back to only one choice daily, as long as you can tolerate it.

Dairy

2 choices daily (organic preferred to eliminate growth-promoters/ hormones/antibiotics).

¼ cup part-skim ricotta cheese, 1 oz. part-skim mozzarella cheese, 1 oz. goat cheese or ¼ cup crumbled, 1 small cup (1/2 cup) organic unsweetened yogurt (may sweeten with Stevia/Splenda), OR ½ cup low-fat low-sodium cottage cheese (lower in calories and fat than most cheeses and a good source of protein).

Note: Most cheeses have high fat content and are high in cholesterol and sodium, therefore are not considered a healthy disease-preventative food choice. Be sure to read labels; know exactly what you are eating! Caution, if constipation, diarrhea, bloating, or excess phlegm occurs, eliminate dairy.

Remember only one dairy serving per meal. Don't double up.

Eggs

1 daily.

(This adjustment is needed because of the reintroduction of dairy, which is high in fat, but also a good protein source).

Nuts

½ oz. daily. (To be used in place of egg snack.)

½ oz. almonds (12 whole almonds – helps prevent heart disease and lowers cholesterol; also a good source of vitamin E, copper, magnesium, good fats and protein) or walnuts (walnuts- good source of EFA linoleic and alpha-linoeic acids, they also contain a powerful antioxidant called ellagic acid that's known to fight cancer cells; are chock full of selenium, zinc, vitamin E and iron).

NOTE: Remember to have nuts in place of hard boiled egg snack.

Animal Protein Sources

Same as before.

Fats

1 tablespoon + 2 teaspoons daily.

1 tablespoon flaxseed oil, and 2 teaspoons of olive oil daily. (To compensate for the added dairy fat. If you choose NOT to add in second dairy choice, then allow 2 tablespoons daily, as before.)

Alcohol

Same as before.

OR

1– low carb or light beer may substitute added carb/starch 2-3 times weekly.

Sugar

Same as before.

Spices

Same as before.

Considerations

Breakfast can now have 4 meal choices: 1 egg with 1 slice of Ezekiel toast with ¼ cup ricotta cheese spread on it- topped with 3 peach slices or ¼ cup of fruit of choice, OR 1½ packets or ½ cup (dry before cooked) oatmeal or oat bran (higher fiber content) sweetened with Stevia or Splenda + 2 tablespoons of unsweetened soy milk + ½ cup of unsweetened applesauce with cinnamon (to be eaten after the grain to level out blood sugar levels; counts as 1/2 fruit serving.) OR ½ cup of yogurt with 1 serving of fruit, and 1 slice of Ezekiel bread drizzled with flaxseed oil. These are the choices to alternate with the breakfast smoothie every other day.

NOTE: Spend your new carb choices wisely; and consume fruit at the end of the meal to regulate blood sugar levels.

Continue exercising 30 minutes 3-5 times weekly.

If weight loss continues, you can now begin the final two weeks of the program. If weight loss was hindered during this segment, then you will hold at weeks 5 and 6 until weight loss begins again. You may have to cut back on 1 dairy and 1 carb choice (week 5) or add more exercise to your plan to compensate for the additional calories. Weeks 7 and 8 are maintenance weeks. You can still continue to lose weight, but this segment will teach you how to add in other foods without gaining weight back, and how to maintain your weight loss once you have reached your goal.

Chapter Six

Segment Four, The Balancing Act

You are about to begin the final segment of this program. Congratulations on your success thus far. You have not only lost weight, but you have accomplished something far greater. You have acted responsibly by taking control of your health! In the past six weeks you have detoxified your body and given it the necessary fuel to thrive, stacking the odds in your favor to ward off disease. As I've mentioned before, this program was designed to boost your own natural defenses; and by doing so your body will be ready to fight viruses, bacterial infections and chronic disease. You are building a fortress that is guarded by an undefeatable army called your immune system.

In this segment you will incorporate additional foods like butter, all-fruit jams, meatloaf, chicken parmesan, desserts, as well as additional food choices. I will also help you overcome weight-loss challenges like dining out, going to the movies or to parties, and teach you how to say NO politely. You will continue to be educated on the importance of balance for the continued success of weight loss or weight maintenance. So let's get started.

One of the many perks of this program, or as I like to refer to as pleasant side effects, is regaining cognitive function. Loss of cognitive function is anything to do with our thinking skills such as, memory loss, forgetfulness, not being able to recall something we know when we need it most, and plain ole mental fog. The FED program gives this function back to us as it peels away layers of toxins, metals, and waste. This resurrection will help us greatly in our everyday lives, especially during this segment. One of the many ways it will come in handy is when you are away from home on either business or pleasure. Your hardest task will be to remember and keep track of the food you consume. This is when you'll recall from your memory banks this eight-week program and all you've learned. Keeping a mental tally, or a journal to list everything you consume, including beverages, is vital to the success of continued weight loss or maintenance. Journaling is great when you find you have a hectic itinerary and may miss meals or snacks. This is where you'll get into trouble. Eating off track throws us off balance, especially our blood sugar levels. It is imperative to plan ahead before you go on vacation or on that business trip, exactly what, where, and when your meals will be. It will be a little more work on your part, but will save you greatly in the end. Recently my family and I went on a cruise and my main concern was gaining weight. Everyone I spoke to that had sailed before, complained about how much weight they had gained; so I planned ahead. I called the travel agency and told them that I was "food challenged" and needed to know what kinds of food would be served and when. They laughed initially, until they discovered I was serious, and then quickly changed their tune and were very accommodating. I was able to get the cruise line's website so that I could go online to see their menus and their hours of operation for the cafés and restaurants. I discovered that I could even request fresh fruit in the room for snacking. I am happy to say that I thoroughly enjoyed myself during my first sailing and I even lost two pounds. As I said planning ahead pays off. Cruising, by the way, is a great way to escape, have fun, and stay active. There are so many activities and tons of walking between decks. Planning ahead is the key to keeping yourself in balance, especially when away from home.

The next challenge is dining out. This challenge probably has the easiest fix. When dining out always know your destination so once again you can plan ahead. I have actually called the restaurant to make sure there was something on the menu that I could eat. If there was not, then I would change my plans. When seated at the table, have the waiter place the bread and butter on the other side of the table. These breads are generally the kinds of bread that are nutritionally void and do nothing but aggravate the digestive tract. If you are alone or with a friend that shares your dietary preferences, ask the waiter to skip the bread and bring the salads right out…a caution though about the salad portion of the meal: this is where a lot of dieters make a huge mistake. Hold the bacon, cheese, croutons, and most of importantly- the dressing, and always bring your own salad dressing. I have been doing this for years. I have a small container that's similar to a small baby food jar, which would also work just fine. If you forget your own dressing, then the only option is vinegar and oil. You can also order your entrée any way you please and most places are very happy to oblige. I have actually walked out of a few places that were not accommodating; and I must admit I made no bones about showing my displeasure. Order poultry, fish, or lean meat, broiled or grilled, blackened or Cajun style, dry (which simply means plain), or pan seared.

Avoid fried, baked (because of hidden sauces), and breaded foods. Ask the waiter if you're not sure about a selection. Side items should include vegetables, but first ask what they are and how they are prepared. A small yam, sweet potato, **or** corn on the cob is also an allowable choice, however, remember the food combining rules: no grain/carbs with proteins at meals and only one vegetable/carb. I'm afraid there's not much to do about the dessert, even the fruit is usually soaked in syrup or else they are high glycemic fruits. I usually will let someone else order a dessert, like my husband, and then have a taste but only if I absolutely have to. If I do splurge on a sample then I immediately swish water around my mouth to neutralize the acid from the sugar. Lemon water would be even better. The idea is to also get the taste out of your mouth as soon as possible. I truly believe that sugar is an addiction and best avoided.

Finally, the last challenge I will discuss is going out. Whether it is going to the movies or a party, it is pretty much the same fix. Make sure you eat plenty of food BEFORE you leave the house. This serves two purposes. The first is so you won't be hungry when you arrive at your destination and the second is so you can refuse fattening appetizers or desserts by giving the excuse that you just ate. If the affair is scheduled during your eating time, try to find out what is being served. If it is something you can work into your program, then enjoy, if it is not, then eat ahead of time and just pick at the meal eating only what you can so you don't offend your hostess. Also practice saying the words *NO THANK YOU.* There are many people whose sole purpose in life is to push food. Food pushers don't like to take no for an answer, but be firm and stick to your guns. Going to the movies is something my husband and I enjoy doing. I always bring my own snack. I usually bring a sliced apple with cinnamon or fresh cherries (when in season), or dried apricots. These are sweet snacks that will satisfy my sweet tooth and fit nicely into a zip-lock bag.

This covers the weight loss challenges, however, keep in mind that we are all human. At any given time, we should do the best that we can at that time. Some times are going to be better and easier than others, and that's okay.

Now that you're ready to move on to maintenance let's begin.

FAT ELIMINATION AND DETOX PROGRAM
Segment 4/Week 7

Supplements

Same as before.

*Digestive Enzymes: Digest Gold by Enzymedica as directed.

*Probiotics: Nature's Way Primadophilis

(I highly recommend incorporating probiotics (friendly bacteria) into your diet on a daily basis. 'Nature's Way Primadophilis' is a good, once-a-day probiotic. Health benefits include: assists in digestion, inhibits pathogenic organisms in the digestive tract, has antifungal properties, aids immune function, and enhances absorption of nutrients).

Beverages

*8 oz. warm water with ½ squeezed lemon in a.m. and p.m.

*2 oz. unsweetened cranberry juice with 6 oz. clean filtered water 2 times daily.

*4-8oz. glasses of clean-filtered water daily. Can include 1 cup of decaffeinated tea (green or herbal preferred.)

*1 cup of decaffeinated coffee in the a.m., if necessary (does not count toward water intake).

Beverages such as soda (diet and regular) are not healthy choices because of artificial sweeteners and high fructose corn syrup. Carbonated water like Perrier, Pellegrino, seltzer, or club soda are acceptable beverages, however, a steady diet of them would not be good for digestion. Pure fruit juices with no added sugar can be consumed sparingly and only in 4 oz. increments and must be substituted for a fruit serving. Pineapple juice is very high on the glycemic chart, so it is best to avoid it or use it sparingly. Since you have already been without caffeine for 7 weeks it is best to stay caffeine free. Caffeine has contributed to many health problems. Decaffeinated coffee and green and herbal teas are permitted sweetened only with Stevia or Splenda.

Vegetables

8-10 cups/10-12 cups/ 12-14 cups daily (depending on BMR)

Same as before but you may add in once daily ½ cup peas, edamame (soybeans are a rich source of phytoestrogens, a weaker version of the hormone estrogen we produce naturally, that helps to keep raging estrogen in check; normalizing levels.), ½ ear of corn (high glycemic; use sparingly), ½ cup winter squash, or a small 5-6 oz. yam (excellent source of fiber and beta-carotene), ½ cup of black or pinto beans (these high protein and high-fiber, disease-fighting legumes are great tossed in salads in place of chicken or fish, or as a condiment to an egg breakfast (do not consume with any other protein sources because it impedes digestion). Benefits are numerous: lowers cholesterol, protects against cancer and heart disease, and helps stabilize blood sugar levels).

Parsnips, white potatoes, red-skinned potatoes, pumpkin, sweet potatoes, and beets are all high glycemic vegetables and should be avoided except for the rare occasion or holiday when they are served. White potatoes, rate right up there with glucose. Corn and yam are also higher up on the glycemic chart but can be used 2-3 times per week. All others are acceptable. When consuming vegetables, keep in mind that the more vivid the color, the more nutrient dense it is. Choose lorraine, raddichio, endive, or chickory over iceberg for your lettuce choice; and be sure to include plenty of cruciferous vegetables like cabbage, broccoli, brussel sprouts, and cauliflower. These are the vegetables of choice for cancer prevention and for fighting cancer.

Note: Work these new vegetable choices in as part of your vegetable allowances, not in addition to.

Fruits

3 servings daily. Same as before + you may add in:

½ banana, small bunch of grapes, 1 cup melon, or 4 oz. orange juice, 2-3 times weekly as 1 serving of fruit. (high glycemic fruit, use sparingly).

Fruit should be used sparingly because of fructose (sugar) content. Choose preferred fruits as mentioned throughout the program over higher glycemic choices like pineapple, raisins, dried dates, watermelon, and cantaloupe. Choose fresh or frozen and avoid canned or pre-packaged because of additives and preservatives.

Grains

Twice daily.

Add in ½ cup brown rice, OR ½ cup (dry before cooked) oatmeal or oatbran (higher fiber) or 1 ½ packets, no sodium only (oats have powerful compounds called saponins, which bind to and eliminate cholesterol and cholesterol-containing bile) OR 1 slice of Ezekiel low-sodium bread daily. (Good source of protein and fiber).

NOTE: If you have one of the added vegetables for this segment, do not combine them at the same meal as your grain choice: 1 vegetable starch and 1 grain choice at separate meals daily. Also note how your body feels. Determine if the second added carb is causing any health problems. If so, then decrease back to only one choice daily as long as you can tolerate it. Do not have meat/fish protein with grain/carb at the same meal; they do not combine well for digestion.

Too many carbohydrates gunk up the works and slow metabolism, not to mention promotes Candida Albicans. Avoid all processed grains like cakes, cookies, pancakes, waffles, white bread and most commercial breads, pasta, and cereals. Include high protein/fiber choices such as, sprouted grains, brown rice, oats, wheat bran, and whole grain cereals without added sugar.

Dairy

2 choices daily (organic preferred, to eliminate growth-promoters/ hormones/antibiotic).

¼ cup part-skim ricotta cheese, 1 oz. part-skim mozzarella cheese, 1 oz. goat cheese or ¼ cup crumbled, 1 small cup (1/2 cup) organic unsweetened yogurt (may sweeten with Stevia/Splenda), *or*, ½ cup low-fat low-sodium cottage cheese (lower in calories and fat than most cheeses and a good source of protein).

NOTE: Caution, if constipation, diarrhea, bloating, or excess phlegm occurs, eliminate dairy. Remember only one dairy serving per meal. Do NOT double up.

Be careful when consuming dairy products as most are a high source of saturated fat. Choose soy cheeses or almond cheese, Soy Dream instead of ice cream (only on special occasions because of sugar content), and substitute soy milk instead of regular milk whenever possible.

Eggs

1 daily.

(This adjustment is needed because of the reintroduction of dairy, which is high in fat, but also a good protein source).

Nuts

½ oz. daily (to be used in the place of egg snack).

½ oz. almonds (12 whole almonds help prevent heart disease and lower cholesterol; also a good source of vitamin E, copper, magnesium, good fats and protein) or walnuts (12 walnut halves are a good source of EFA linoleic and alpha-linoeic acids, they also contain a powerful antioxidant called ellagic acid that's known to fight cancer cells; are chock full of selenium, zinc, vitamin E and iron)

Animal Protein Sources

Same as before.

Fats

1 tablespoon + 2 teaspoons daily.

1 tablespoon flaxseed oil, and 2 teaspoons of olive oil daily.

NOTE: To compensate for the added dairy fat. If you choose NOT to add in second dairy choice, then allow 2 tablespoons daily, as before.

One tablespoon of flaxseed oil will remain the constant for oil throughout the program and is recommended to continue through maintenance. The second fat choice can include split up into 3 teaspoons using: unsalted organic butter, ghee (clarified butter), or olive oil. It is imperative to keep fat value at roughly 30 percent of the diet. So be careful not to over do it on dairy and fats. Keep track of what you are eating.

Alcohol

Same as before.

OR

1- Low carb or light beer may substitute added carb/starch 2-3 times weekly.

Sugar

Same as before.

Sugar (as I've stated before) feeds and breeds disease. If you must have something that contains sugar, make sure you also consume foods or supplements that will regulate blood sugar. Probiotics are a must here because sugar also feeds Candida Albicans, yeast. You can bake your own desserts using natural sweeteners like applesauce, Stevia, rice syrup, or barley malt. Maple syrup is too high in sugars so it is best to avoid it. Use unsweetened, melted, fruit preserves, instead. I will include a few delicious recipes using these sweeteners in the recipe section.

Spices

Same as before.

Spice it up and enjoy the many different combinations of spices available!

Considerations

Breakfast can now consist of 4 meal choices: 1 egg with 1 slice of Ezekiel toast with ¼ cup ricotta cheese spread on it. You can sprinkle on a little Stevia for a sweeter taste with 3 peach slices or ¼ cup of fruit of choice, OR, 1½ packets or ½ cup (dry before cooked) oatmeal or oat bran (higher fiber content) sweetened with Stevia or Splenda + 2 tablespoons of unsweetened soy milk + ½ cup of unsweetened applesauce with cinnamon (to be eaten after the grain to level out blood sugar levels; counts as ½ fruit serving), OR ½ cup of yogurt with 1 serving of fruit, and 1 slice of Ezekiel bread drizzled with flaxseed oil. These are the choices to alternate with the breakfast smoothie every other day.

Remember: Spend your new carb choices wisely, and consume fruit at the end of the meal to regulate blood sugar levels.

Continue exercising 30-45 minutes 3-5 times weekly.
Congratulations! You now move into the final week!!

FAT ELIMINATION AND DETOX PROGRAM
Segment 4/Final Week

This final week is the same as week 7 as far as structure goes, however a few more foods have been added in. Be sure to read through the entire program. There is also a sample menu for the maintenance program for week 8. After this point, you graduate on to eating at your own pace. I strongly recommend that you use all the knowledge you've gained thus far to plan your meals, making good healthy food choices for disease prevention.

Supplements

Same as before.

*Digestive Enzymes - Digest Gold by Enzymedica as directed. (I recommend these, especially in this segment with the reintroduction of dairy. Dairy is difficult for many people to digest, therefore, digestive enzymes will aid in the digestion process).

*Probiotics - I highly recommend incorporating probiotics (friendly bacteria) into your diet on a daily basis. Nature's Way Primadophilis is a good once a day probiotic. Health benefits include: assists in digestion, inhibits pathogenic organisms in the digestive tract, has antifungal properties, aids immune function, and enhances absorption of nutrients).

*Calcium/magnesium - with vitamin D complex by Country Life 2-4 capsules daily, especially for women, or Calcium/Magnesium by Floradix (this particular blend is a liquid and is one of the best products for maximum absorption and is essential for bone health, menopausal symptoms or PMS, aids with constipation, and also reduces heart irregularity).

Beverages

*8 oz. warm water with ½ squeezed lemon in a.m. and p.m.

*2 oz. unsweetened cranberry juice with 6 oz. clean filtered water 2 times daily.

*4-8 oz. glasses of clean filtered water daily. Can include 1 cup of decaffeinated tea (green or herbal preferred).

*1cup of decaffeinated coffee in the a.m. (if necessary) does not count toward water intake.

Beverages such as soda (diet and regular) are not healthy choices because of artificial sweeteners and high fructose corn syrup. Carbonated water like Perrier, Pellegrino, seltzer, or club soda are acceptable beverages, however, a steady diet of them would not be good for digestion. Pure fruit juices with no added sugar can be consumed sparingly and only in 4 oz. increments and must be substituted for a fruit serving. Pineapple juice is very high on the glycemic chart, so it is best to avoid it or use it sparingly. Since you have already been without caffeine for 7 weeks it is best to stay caffeine free. Caffeine has contributed to many health problems. Decaffeinated coffee and green and herbal teas are permitted sweetened only with Stevia or Splenda.

Vegetables

8-10 cups/10-12 cups/ 12-14 daily (depending on BMR).

Same as before but you may add one of the following once daily: ½ cup peas, edamame (soybeans are a rich source of phytoestrogens, a weaker version of the hormone estrogen we produce naturally, that helps to keep raging estrogen in check; normalizing levels.), ½ ear of corn (high glycemic; use sparingly), ½ cup winter squash, or a small yam or ½ of a small sweet potato (excellent source of fiber and beta-carotene), ½ cup of black or pinto beans (these high-protein and high-fiber, disease-fighting legumes are great tossed in salads in place of chicken or fish, or as a condiment to an egg breakfast. Do not consume this with any other protein sources; impedes digestion. Benefits are numerous: lowers cholesterol, protects against cancer and heart disease and helps stabilize blood sugar levels).

NOTE: Work these new vegetable choices in as part of your vegetable allowances not in addition to.

Fruits

3 servings daily. Same as before + you may add in:

¼ cantaloupe, ½ cup pineapple, 1 cup watermelon, a small box or a ½ oz. of raisins 2-3 times weekly as 1 serving of fruit. (Caution, the high glycemic fruit should be used sparingly).

Fruit should be used sparingly because of fructose (sugar) content. Choose preferred fruits as mentioned throughout the program over higher glycemic choices like pineapple, raisins, dried dates, watermelon, and cantaloupe. Use these added fruit choices sparingly. Choose fresh or frozen and avoid canned or pre-packaged because of additives and preservatives.

Grains

Twice daily.

Add in ½ cup brown rice, or oatmeal or oat bran (higher fiber) 1 ½ packets - no sodium only (oats have powerful compounds called saponins, which bind to and eliminate cholesterol and cholesterol-containing bile) or 1 slice of Ezekiel low-sodium bread daily. (Good source of protein and fiber).

NOTE: If you have one of the added vegetables for this segment, then do not combine them at the same meal as your grain choice, 1 vegetable starch and 1 grain choice at separate meals daily). Also note how your body feels. Determine if the second added carb is causing any health problems. If so, then decrease back to only one choice daily as long as you can tolerate it.

Too many carbohydrates can gunk up the works and slow metabolism, not to mention promotes Candida Albicans. Avoid all processed grains like cakes, cookies, pancakes, waffles, white bread and most commercial breads, pasta, and cereals. Pasta should only be consumed once in awhile and never combine with meat. Include high protein/fiber choices such as, sprouted grains, brown rice, oats, wheat bran, and whole grain cereals without added sugar.

Dairy

2 choices daily (organic preferred, to eliminate growth-promoters/ hormones/antibiotics).

¼ cup part-skim ricotta cheese, 1 oz. part-skim mozzarella cheese, goat cheese, 1 small cup (1/2 cup) organic unsweetened yogurt (may sweeten with Stevia/Splenda). (Health benefits for yogurt are due to the friendly bacteria, Lactobacillus acidophilus, which protects against gastrointestinal yeast and urinary tract infections; also strengthens the immune system), or ½ cup low-fat low-sodium cottage cheese (lower in calories and fat than most cheeses and a good source of protein).

Watch out for dairy/milk products as most are a high source of saturated fat. Choose soy cheeses or almond cheese, Soy Dream instead of ice cream (only on special occasions), and substitute soy milk instead of regular milk whenever possible.

Eggs

1 daily.

(This adjustment is needed because of the reintroduction of dairy, which is high in fat, but also a good protein source).

Nuts

½ oz. daily. (To be a substitute for the egg snack.)

½ oz. almonds (12 whole almonds- helps prevent heart disease and lowers cholesterol; also a good source of vitamin E, copper, magnesium, good fats and protein), or walnuts (12 walnut halves- good source of EFA's linoleic and alpha-linoeic acids; they also contain a powerful antioxidant called ellagic acid that's known to fight cancer cells; are chock full of selenium, zinc, vitamin E and iron), in place of hard boiled egg snack.

Animal Protein Sources

Same as before.

Fats

1 tablespoon + 2 teaspoons daily.

1 tablespoon flaxseed oil, and 2 teaspoons of olive oil daily.

NOTE: To compensate for the added dairy fat. If you choose NOT to add in second dairy choice, then allow 2 tablespoons daily, as before.

One tablespoon of flaxseed oil will remain the constant for oil throughout the program and is recommended to continue through maintenance. The second fat choice (split up into 3 teaspoons) can include unsalted organic butter, ghee (clarified butter), or olive oil. It is imperative to keep fat value at roughly 30percent of the diet. So be careful not to overdo it on dairy and fats. Keep track of what you are eating. A lot of programs suggest journaling. If this is something that will help you, I am enclosing a journaling page for your use. After seven weeks on the program however, you should be pretty good at keeping track.

Alcohol

Same as before.

OR

1- Low carb or light beer may substitute added carb/starch 2-3 times weekly.

Use your alcohol choices wisely. Overuse will inhibit your ability to make 'good judgments' and may cause you to make bad food choices, while under the influence. Alcohol is also a sure way to go overboard on your daily caloric intake. It is very high in calories and will add up fast!

Sugar

Same as before.

Sugar as I've stated before feeds and breeds disease. If you must have something that contains sugar, make sure you also consume foods or supplements that will regulate blood sugar. Probiotics are a must here because sugar also feeds Candida Albicans, yeast. You can bake your own desserts using natural sweeteners like applesauce, Stevia, rice syrup, or barley malt. Maple syrup is too high in sugar, so avoid it. Instead use unsweetened fruit preserves melted down. I will include a few delicious recipes using these sweeteners in the recipe section.

Spices

Same as before.

Spice it up and enjoy the many different combinations of spices available!

Considerations

Spend your new carb choices wisely; and consume fruit at the end of the meal to regulate blood sugar levels.

Continue exercising 30-45 minutes 3-5 times weekly.

You will find a sample meal plan for the maintenance program on the following pages. If weight loss was hindered this week, then cut back on added carbs or dairy until weight loss continues.

Good luck and may your new found health continue!

FED Maintenance Sample Menu

(Be sure to add in additional BMR food allowances)

Upon waking: 8 oz. warm water with ½ squeezed lemon.

Breakfast

#1
1 scrambled egg, 1 slice Ezekiel toast w/ 1 teaspoon all fruit jam, ½ cup yogurt sweetened with 1 teaspoon all-fruit jam. 8 oz. cranberry water.

OR

#2
½ cup oat bran (dry before cooking), 1 teaspoon butter, sweetened with Stevia, ¼ cup unsweetened soy milk, ½ cup unsweetened applesauce with cinnamon, or 1 medium apple. 8 oz. cranberry water.

OR

#3
½ cup cottage cheese, ½ serving sliced peaches with cinnamon, 1 slice Ezekiel bread with 1 teaspoon flaxseed oil or butter. 8 oz. cranberry water.

OR

#4
Fruit smoothie made with ¾ cup unsweetened soy milk, 1 scoop protein powder, 1 cup fruit, Stevia, dash of cinnamon.

All of these breakfast choices average around 250 calories, 6 grams fat, and 10 grams of protein.

10 a.m. snack - 12 nuts, or fruit

Snack averages 85-90 calories, nuts have added fat so be sure to cut out 1 egg or 1 teaspoon of fat.

Lunch

#1
RAINBOW SALAD

4-8 oz. roasted chicken,
3 cups romaine lettuce
½ cup mushrooms
1 shredded carrot
1 medium tomato sliced,
½ cucumber sliced
½ cup clover sprouts
12 whole green beans
½ sliced yellow pepper,
1 serving Honey Mustard Dressing (minus the honey)
8 oz. Cranberry water

Can sub in 4-8 oz. turkey or grilled fish.

OR

#2
TUNA SALAD

4-8 oz. low sodium canned chunk light tuna (or sardines)
bed of lettuce, tomatoes, sprouts, cucumbers,
1 serving dressing, 1 hard boiled egg. 8 oz. Cranberry water.

OR

#3
GRILLED SALMON/CHICKEN

4-8 oz. grilled salmon or chicken, side salad, small baked yam drizzled with 1 teaspoon flaxseed oil or butter w/ cinnamon. 8 oz. cranberry water.

All three choices for lunch average 300 calories, 11 grams of fat, and 25-30 grams of protein.

2 p.m. – 16 oz. water beverage

4 p.m. snack – hard boiled egg or fruit.

Snack averages 70-90 calories.

Dinner

#1
TURKEY MEATLOAF

4-8 oz. turkey meatloaf, steamed broccoli w/ lemon and 1 teaspoon flaxseed oil, Small yam with 1 teaspoon butter with cinnamon. 8 oz. cranberry water.

OR

#2
PAN-SEARED SNAPPER

4-8 oz. pan-seared snapper Cajun style, stir-fry vegetables,

(Bok choy, 1 carrot, snow peas, water chestnuts, sweet onion,) sautéed in 1 teaspoon olive oil with water to cover bottom of pan, sliced corn on the cob, 1 teaspoon of garlic butter. 8 oz. cranberry water.

OR

#3
CHICKEN PARMESAN

Chicken Parmesan, (w/1 cup sodium free tomato sauce, ¼ cup soy mozzarella cheese, spices), 1cup sautéed, fresh spinach, baby bella mushrooms and fresh elephant garlic, small side salad (2 cups), with Italian style dressing.

Recipe: (use half)

(1 tablespoon flaxseed oil, 1 tablespoon apple cider vinegar, 1 tablespoon water, basil, oregano, garlic, Stevia)

8 oz. Cranberry water.

All three choices for dinner average 550 calories, 13 grams of fat, and 30 grams protein.

8 p.m. snack – ½ serving fruit w/ ½ cup yogurt sweetened with Stevia or Chocolate Cherries Jubilee Gelato (see recipe in Chapter 7). 8 oz. herb tea w/ lemon.

Macronutrient Totals

Daily average for calories is 1400, fat grams are 41-45, protein grams are 70-75, carbohydrates are 175-180 grams, and fiber is 30-35 grams. Macronutrient breakdown is:

Fat= 30 percent
Protein= 20 percent
Carbohydrates=50 percent

These totals are for those with a lower BMR consuming 4 oz. of protein daily. Those eating at the higher BMR level (6 oz.) are as follows:

Daily average for calories is 1800, fat grams are 55-58, protein grams are 110-115, carbohydrate grams are 200, and fiber 33-37. Macronutrient breakdown is:

Fat=30 percent
Protein= 25 percent
Carbohydrates=45 percent

Highest BMR level (8oz.) is as follows:

Daily average for calories is 2200, fat grams are 73-75, protein grams are 133-137, carbohydrate grams are 245, and fiber 37-40 grams. Macronutrient breakdown is:

Fat=30 percent
Protein=25 percent
Carbohydrates=45 percent

It is imperative to keep these percentages throughout your weight loss journey, or at least until you've dropped your BMR to the lower level. Balance is the whole key to successful weight loss program. It is of vital importance to remember NOT to over exercise as this drastically upsets these percentages, making them insufficient. If you have reached your goal and want to maintain your weight, then you must add in more choices until you stop losing weight. Be careful to add food choices in balance. For example, try adding in two ounces of protein, 1 teaspoon of fat, and 1 grain/carb or 1 dairy choice. This will give you an extra 180-200 calories per day. This should help you to maintain your new weight. You can always fall back to individual weeks if you start gaining again, until you reach your desired goal and are able to successfully maintain that weight.

Chapter Seven

FED Recipes, For A Healthier Life

Now that you have mastered the FED program, I have included a variety of healthy recipes for you to incorporate into your everyday life. These are quick, easy recipes that were created for everyone, even the complete novice, when it comes to cooking. There is also a glossary of cooking terms at the end of this chapter for your convenience. I have selected recipes for breakfast, lunch, dinner, and desserts as well. These recipes are also lower carbohydrate choices, to help keep weight from creeping back up. Always remember the key to successful weight management is balance.

The cooking techniques used in these recipes are very basic. I steam vegetables by either using a steamer basket, or a saucepan with just enough water to cover the bottom of the pan; then place vegetables in the pan cover and steam until done. Steaming times can vary depending on the vegetables, but I generally steam for three to ten minutes. Stir frying is another quick and easy method for cooking vegetables. I spray a frying pan or wok with olive oil spray, then use 1 teaspoon of olive oil and a little water in the pan; add vegetables (the longer cooking ones first, like carrots, onions or cauliflower), cover the pan and let cook for a few minutes; then remove lid and stir-fry until tender. Be careful not to overcook vegetables because you will lose valuable nutrients.

As previously mentioned you will also want to include plenty of raw vegetables as well, so you can gain the many health benefits of the vegetable's enzymes. I eat a large raw vegetable salad at least five to six times weekly, especially in the warmer months. In the cooler months I prefer stir-frying or I'll lightly steam vegetables, so that I retain their health properties. Rule of thumb is if they are still crunchy, then you have retained the nutrients and the enzymes. Oftentimes if I feel cold, the last thing I want to do is to eat a cold salad, so instead I grill chicken or fish, and top my salad with it while it is still hot, then dress the salad with warm salad dressing. You can warm dressings made with flaxseed oil, however, only warm them slightly to avoid damaging the oil. It also helps to bring vegetables to room temperature in the cool months before consuming them.

Meats are usually pan-seared, fried in a small amount of olive or canola oil, or grilled. Always rinse meat or fish under cool water then pat dry before cooking. Don't forget to use seasonings liberally. You can spray olive oil directly on top of the meat, or fish before seasoning. This enables the seasoning to adhere better. Refer back to chapter four if you need to be reminded of the many medicinal properties of spices.

Organic items like produce, spices, dairy products, and meat, are still highly recommended. You must continue to support your liver and other vital organs by protecting them from pesticides and other possible contaminants. As I have stated numerous times in this book, YOU ARE WHAT YOU EAT. If you have trouble finding organic foods in your area, just speak to the manager of your local grocery store. They are usually very happy to accommodate their customers. I have also included a few mail order organic companies in the resource section for your convenience.

MAIN DISH RECIPES

PAN-SEARED FISH/CHICKEN

12 oz. white fish of choice or Springer Mountain Farms chicken (cod, mahi, snapper, haddock, halibut, scallops, shrimp)

Cajun seasoning or seasonings of choice

Canola spray/olive oil spray

Preparations:

Rinse fish/chicken in cool water and pat dry. Spray skillet lightly with canola spray. Place fish/chicken in hot pan sprayed with oil spray and lightly spray tops of fish with canola spray. Liberally apply spices. Press fish/chicken with spatula down into pan and sear for approximately 30 seconds then flip fish/chicken and apply spices again. Cover and simmer until done. (Times will vary depending on thickness.) Makes 2 six oz. servings or 3 four oz. servings.

PIZZA FISH

12 oz. cod or haddock

1 cup tomato sauce or stewed diced tomatoes

2 teaspoons of olive oil

Pinch of basil, oregano, and garlic seasonings

½ cup soy veggie shreds (soy mozzarella cheese) or rice mozzarella cheese

Preparations:

Heat skillet with 2 teaspoons of oil. Place fish in hot pan and pan fry 10 minutes on each side, or until done. Add tomatoes or sauce and seasonings, over the tops of the fish, and top with cheese. Cover and let simmer for 10 minutes until cheese is melted. Serve with wilted spinach with garlic and lemon. Makes 2 six oz. servings or 3 four oz. servings.

NOTE: Can substitute in chicken for fish to make chicken parmesan.

SAVORY TURKEY MEATLOAF

16 oz. Shelton's ground turkey
2 egg whites
Savory, Parsley and Thyme, seasonings
½ small onion, minced
OR
1 teaspoon dried minced onion

Preparations:

Mix ground turkey and the rest of the ingredients together in a bowl. Then form loaf and place in a mini-loaf pan sprayed with canola/olive oil. Bake in a 375 degree oven for 30 minutes, or until done. Makes 4 servings.

ZUCCHINI BOATS

2 large size zucchini

1 bag frozen vegetable mix of broccoli, cauliflower, carrots, water chestnuts, and soy beans (or any combo will do)

8 oz. ground Shelton's turkey

½ teaspoon garlic powder

1 cup soy veggie shreds (mozzarella cheese) almond, or rice cheese.

olive oil spray

Preparations:

Cut tops off zucchini and slice in half lengthwise. Place in pot of boiling water and boil until tender. Remove from water and let drain a few minutes until cool enough to handle. Steam frozen vegetables for 10 minutes. Scoop seeds-pulp from center of zucchini and set pulp aside. Combine steamed vegetables, mashed up zucchini pulp, cheese, and garlic powder and set aside. Brown the turkey in fry pan and while hot add to vegetable mixture. Toss until cheese starts to melt. Fill zucchini halves as full as possible. Place in Pyrex baking dish sprayed with olive oil spray and bake at 350 degrees for 30 minutes, covered loosely with foil. Makes 2 servings.

NOTE: Can add ½ cup tomato sauce + a dash of cayenne to vegetable mixture, for a zesty Spanish influence.

CREAMY CHICKEN DIVAN

8 oz. cooked white meat chicken, sliced
1 package frozen broccoli spears (thawed)
OR
1 package fresh broccoli (steamed)
1 ½ cups low-sodium chicken broth or homemade broth
¼ teaspoon garlic powder
2 tablespoons spelt flour + 2 tablespoons cool water
½ cup veggie cheddar shredds cheese, or almond or rice cheese
olive oil cooking spray

Preparations:

Mix flour with water until smooth. Heat broth to a low boil; add flour mixture and stir until thickened. Remove from heat stir in garlic. Spray an 8x8 pan with cooking spray. Evenly distribute broccoli spears in the bottom pan and place chicken on top. Pour gravy over the top and top with cheese. Cover with foil and bake in a 350 degree oven for 30 minutes. Makes 2 servings.

STUFFEDPEPPERS

2 green organic peppers
2 cups brown rice
1 cup tomato sauce
½ sweet onion, diced
1 8oz. package goat cheese crumbles
½ teaspoon garlic powder
1 tablespoon olive oil

Preparations:

Cut peppers in half and scoop seeds. Steam until tender. Prepare rice as directed. Sauté onion in sauté pan in a small amount of water until tender or water evaporates. Add in rice, ½ the cheese, ½ the tomato sauce, garlic and olive oil. Blend with spatula. Take four pepper halves and stuff with filling. Place in sprayed Pyrex baking dish. Top each half with remaining sauce and cheese. Bake at 350, covered with foil, for 30 minutes. Makes 2 servings.

NOTE: If you want this recipe to be a higher protein choice, omit 1 cup of rice and add 8 oz. of ground beef or turkey.

HOMEMADE TOMATO SAUCE

1 large can organic tomato puree + ½ cup water
1 tablespoon olive oil
½ sweet onion (diced)
1 large clove elephant garlic
½ teaspoon dried basil
½ teaspoon dried oregano
sprinkle red pepper flakes
1 packet Stevia/Splenda

Preparations:

Heat oil in skillet and add onion, garlic, and spices. Sauté until tender. Add tomatoes, water, and sweetener. Bring to a slow boil, reduce heat and simmer for 45 minutes. Makes 8- ½ cup servings.

CABBAGE PAN CASSEROLE

1 head Napa cabbage (sliced in half inch slices)
½ sweet onion, sliced
8 oz. ground beef or turkey
1 ½ cups tomato sauce
1 large clove elephant garlic, sliced
½ tablespoon olive oil

Preparations:

Brown meat in a frying pan and set aside. Stir-fry cabbage, onion, and garlic, until tender, using oil and water to cover the bottom of the pan. Add tomato sauce and meat. Simmer, adding water (if necessary) to avoid sticking, for 10 minutes. Makes 2 servings.

STIR-FRYVEGETABLES

½ head napa cabbage (sliced or shredded)
1 sweet onion (sliced)
1 green bell pepper (sliced)
1 red pepper (sliced)
1 carrot (sliced)
1 small can water chestnuts
½ bunch broccoli
1 tablespoon sesame oil
Bragg's Amino-acid spray
Sesame seeds

Preparations:

Place oil in stir-fry pan and heat until hot. Layer vegetables in the order given, except for broccoli. Cover and steam for 5 minutes. Take cover off and stir-fry until tender; add broccoli and cover for 5 minutes longer. Remove from heat and spray Bragg's until vegetables are coated. Sprinkle with sesame seeds and serve. Makes 1 serving.

NOTE: Can add chicken, beef, or fish. Stir-fry meat separately and add to vegetables.

FAVORITE CAJUN SPICE BLEND

½ teaspoon each of the following spices: cayenne, cinnamon, allspice, cloves, garlic powder, onion powder, paprika, ginger, cumin, mustard powder, celery seed, thyme ¼ teaspoon sea salt

Preparations:

Combine all ingredients. Store in an air-tight jar. Shake well before using.

NOTE: This blend is definitely considered a thermogenic blend, which means it raises metabolism.

VEGETABLE SIDE DISHES

TOMATO & ASPARAGUS BAKE

2 tablespoons olive oil
1 pound of fresh asparagus (washed and trimmed)
2 tablespoons chopped celery
2 medium ripe tomatoes (sliced)
½ teaspoon dried basil
½ teaspoon of oregano
½ teaspoon garlic powder
½ cup goat cheese crumbles (low-sodium)

Preparations:

Preheat oven to 350 degrees. Spread oil in the bottom of an 11 x 7 glass pan. Layer asparagus in the bottom of pan and sprinkle with chopped celery. Arrange tomato slices on top (down the center of asparagus) and sprinkle spices and cheese over top. Cover loosely with foil and bake 30 minutes or until asparagus is tender. Makes 4 servings.

FAUX SWEET POTATO CASSEROLE

4 large carrots peeled and sliced
¼ cup unsweetened soy milk
1 tablespoon flaxseed oil
2 tablespoons chopped pecans or walnuts
½ teaspoon cinnamon

Preparations:

Wash, peel, and slice carrots. Steam carrots until tender. Place carrots and remaining ingredients, except nuts, in blender and mix until blended. Stir in or top with nuts and serve. Makes 2 servings.

MASHED CAULIFLOWER

1 organic head cauliflower (cut up)
1 T. flaxseed oil
3 T. unsweetened soy milk
liquid from steaming cauliflower
pinch of lite salt
garlic powder seasoning

Preparations:

Steam cut up cauliflower in a steamer basket or pot, when done reserve liquid for later. Place cauliflower in a food processor or blender, with remaining ingredients. Add reserved liquid from steaming, until desired consistency. Makes 3 or 4 servings.

NOTE: Can also steam ½ sweet onion (sliced), or 1 large clove of elephant garlic (chopped), with cauliflower for a more flavorful dish.

GARLICY GREEN BEANS WITH MUSHROOMS

2 cups fresh green beans (with stems cut off)
1 small container of button or domestic mushrooms (sliced)
1 large clove elephant garlic (sliced)
2 teaspoons olive oil
½ teaspoon garlic powder

Preparations:

Steam green beans and mushrooms. Sautee sliced garlic in oil until brown. Add green beans, mushrooms, and garlic powder and continue sautéing until vegetables are coated with oil and warmed through. Makes 2 servings.

GREENBEAN/CARROT ALMONDINE

4 cups of whole organic green beans
1 carrot, peeled and sliced into 1/8 inch thick slices
1 oz. (24 nuts) whole tamari flavored almonds
1 tablespoon flaxseed oil
½ teaspoon garlic powder

Preparations:

Prepare beans by breaking off stems. Place beans, carrots, and almonds in steamer basket and steam for 5-7 minute only. Remove from pan into glass bowl. Add garlic and flaxseed oil and toss together. For a crunchier recipe, don't steam almonds, add them at the end. Makes 4 servings.

NOTE: This recipe is supposed to be crunchy. The vegetables are just steamed just enough to soften them without depleting them of their vital nutrients. I make a double batch and store it in a container in the refrigerator. It makes a delicious cold salad.

LEMON BROCCOLI

1 large bunch broccoli
½ lemon
1 teaspoon flaxseed oil

Preparations:

Steam broccoli for 5 minutes. Remove from heat and squeeze lemon and drizzle oil over tops of broccoli. Makes 2 servings.

SAUTEED CAJUN MUSHROOMS

1 8-ounce package Mushrooms
2 teaspoons olive oil
½ to 1 teaspoon Favorite Cajun Spice blend (see recipe)

Preparations:

Sautee mushrooms in olive oil and coat with spice blend. Makes 2 servings.

GINGERED CARROTS

4 carrots (peeled and cut)
2 tablespoons pickled ginger (diced)
1 tablespoon canola oil

Preparations:

Steam carrots until tender and set aside. Heat oil in small saucepan, add ginger and sauté for 3 minutes. Add carrots, toss and serve. Makes 2 servings.

SPICED BLACK BEANS

1 can low-sodium black beans
½ sweet onion (diced)
½ cup tomatoes (dices)
½ cup low-sodium chicken broth
1 teaspoon olive oil
1 teaspoon of Favorite Cajun Spice blend

Preparations:

Sauté onion, and tomatoes in broth. Add the rest of the ingredients and simmer 20 minutes. Makes 3 servings.

SWEET POTATO MEDALLIONS

2 medium size sweet potatoes or yams (1/2 inch slices)
1 tablespoon olive oil
Favorite fruit spice blend
¼ cup cherry all-fruit preserves (melted)
cooking spray

Preparations:

Cut ends off sweet potatoes and slice into ½ inch slices. Spray glass pie dish with cooking spray and layer sweet potatoes, brushing each one with oil. Sprinkle spices and drizzle preserves over top. Cover with foil and bake at 350 degrees for 35-40 minutes or until potatoes are tender. Makes 4 servings.

NOTE: This is a great dish to make for the holiday table.

BREAKFAST RECIPES

TRIPLE BERRY PARFAIT

1 cup plain organic yogurt
½ cup blueberries
½ cup strawberries
½ cup blackberries or raspberries
1 packet Stevia

Preparations:

Place ½ cup of blueberries (1/4 cup each) in two dessert parfait cups. Blend Stevia into yogurt. Top blueberries with ¼ cup yogurt in each then add strawberries and top with yogurt; and top off with blackberries or raspberries. (Cherries can also be substituted for one of the berries.) Makes 2 servings.

Note: Layer peaches, raspberries, and nectarines for a variation on this recipe.

FRUITED OATMEAL

1 cup oatmeal (dry before cooking)
2 cups water
1 apple, peeled and diced
1 oz. walnut pieces
½ teaspoon cinnamon
¼ cup unsweetened soy milk
1 packet Stevia

Preparations:

Boil water; stir in oatmeal and apple, and walnuts, simmer 3-5 minutes stirring occasionally. Remove from heat add cinnamon, Stevia and soy milk; cover let stand one minute. Makes 2 servings.

SPANISH OMELETTE

2 eggs, beaten with 1 tablespoon water
¼ sliced onion
½ sliced green pepper
½ cup tomato sauce (low-sodium)
olive oil cooking spray
1 teaspoon parmesan cheese

Preparations:

Sauté onion and pepper until tender, set aside. Spray the bottom of a small frying pan with cooking spray. When hot add egg mixture and sautéed vegetables. Cover and cook until firm. Fold over and add tomato sauce. Remove from heat cover and let stand 1 minute. Top with cheese. Makes 1 serving.

VEGETABLE FRITTATA

4 free roam eggs, beaten with 2 T. water
1 cup of spinach leaves washed and dried OR
¾ cup of frozen spinach, thawed and patted dry
1 cup sliced mushrooms, baby Bella
Canola/olive spray
Seasonings of choice

Sauté spinach and mushrooms in a pan with just enough water to cover the bottom of the pan. Be careful not to burn. When water evaporates remove from heat and transfer to a glass bowl. Rinse pan and spray with canola/olive oil spray. Spread vegetables evenly back in pan and pour eggs over the top. Add seasonings, cover and cook on medium heat until firm. You may flip it carefully if you prefer your eggs well done. Makes 2 servings.

NOTE: You can use any allowable vegetables. This is a good way to get in your leafy greens!

PEPPERS & EGGS

2 eggs
1 green pepper (sliced)
½ small sweet onion (sliced)
1 tablespoon olive oil

Preparations:

Beat eggs and set aside. Sauté peppers and onions, until tender. Add eggs to pan and stir-fry until eggs are done. Makes 1 serving.

BLUEBERRY CINNAMON FRENCH TOAST

4 slices Ezekiel bread (any flavor)
2 large eggs (use 2 egg whites, 1 egg yolk)
½ teaspoon vanilla
½ teaspoon cinnamon
1 packet Stevia/Splenda
1 cup blueberries + ¼ cup water + 1 packet of Stevia/Splenda

Preparations:

Mix eggs, vanilla, cinnamon, and sweetener. Bring blueberries and water and sweetener to a slow boil, cover and simmer 10 minutes. Dip each slice of Ezekiel bread in egg mixture and place in a pre-heated frying pan sprayed with canola oil cooking spray. Pan fry both sides until slightly brown. Top with blueberry syrup. Makes 2 servings.

SPROUTED SPICED FRENCH TOAST

2 slices sprouted grain bread
1 egg (beaten)
2 tablespoons soy milk
Pinch of favorite fruit blend
½ teaspoon vanilla
2 tablespoons all-fruit preserves (melted)
Cooking spray

Preparations:

Place egg, milk, vanilla, and spices in bowl and beat. Dip bread (both sides) into mixture and pan fry with canola oil cooking spray flipping bread once. Drizzle with melted preserves. Makes 1 serving.

PUMPKIN/AGAVE MUFFINS

1 cup pumpkin + ½ cup agave nectar sweetener
1 egg
¼ cup melted canoleo or olive oil margarine
½ cup unsweetened soy milk + ¼ cup water
1 cup soy flour
½ cup oat flour + ½ cup dry oats
1/ ½ teaspoons pumpkin pie spice
2 teaspoons baking powder + 1 teaspoon baking soda
½ teaspoons salt (optional)

Preparations:

Mix dry ingredients. Mix wet ingredients (batter). Slowly add wet batter to dry ingredients. Blend well then, spoon into mini-muffin pans and bake at 350 for 15 minutes. (You can sprinkle dry oats or pumpkin seeds on top of batter, before baking.) Makes 18 mini-muffins.

SALAD DRESSING RECIPES

GREEK STYLE DRESSING

1 tablespoon olive oil
1 tablespoon apple cider vinegar
1 tablespoon water
2 tablespoons feta or goat cheese (crumbled fine)
1 tablespoon chopped green olives (about 3)
1/8 teaspoon dried basil
dash of red pepper flakes

Preparations:

Mix all ingredients in a shaker container with lid and shake vigorously until blended. Makes 1 serving.

HONEY MUSTARD DRESSING(minus the honey)

1 tablespoon Dijon mustard (Wheat Free)
1 tablespoon apple-cider vinegar
1 tablespoon flaxseed oil
½ packet Stevia/Splenda

Preparations:

Mix all ingredients in container with lid. Shake vigorously. Makes 1 serving.

SWEET ITALIAN DRESSING

1 tablespoon olive oil
1 tablespoon apple-cider vinegar
1 tablespoon water
1/8 teaspoon each of basil, oregano, and garlic powder
½ packet Stevia

Preparations:

Mix all ingredients in container with lid. Shake vigorously. Makes 1 serving.

NOTE: You can use any of your favorite spices in this recipe and I've even added 2 tablespoons of grated Romano cheese and red pepper flakes for an added zing.

CREAMY CUCUMBER DRESSING

½ cucumber, peeled
1 tablespoon flaxseed oil
2 tablespoons unsweetened soy milk
dash of dill and garlic powder
½ packet Stevia

Preparations:

Blend all ingredients in blender until well blended. Makes 1 serving.

ZESTY MUSTARD VINEGRETTE

¼ cup olive oil
¼ cup apple cider vinegar
¼ cup water
¼ teaspoon dried basil
¼ teaspoon oregano
pinch garlic salt
1 teaspoon grey poupon mustard
1 packet Stevia/Splenda

Preparations:

Place all ingredients in a shaker bottle and shake well. For best results refrigerate overnight. Makes 6 servings of 2 tablespoons each.

LUNCH RECIPES

RAINBOW SALAD

4-6 oz. roasted chicken
3 cups romaine lettuce
½ cup mushrooms
1 shredded carrot
I medium tomato sliced
½ cucumber slice
½ cup clover sprouts
12 whole green beans
1 slice yellow pepper

Preparations:

Layer vegetables in order given. Place roasted chicken on top. Serve with dressing suggestions below. Makes 1 serving.

NOTE: You can also use grilled fish, canned low-sodium tuna or sardines.

FAUX CHICKEN WINGS

1 pkg. Springer Mountain Farms Thin chicken cutlets
2 tablespoons olive oil
cayenne pepper
Cajun spice blend recipe
Honey mustard dressing, minus the honey

Preparations:

Rinse and cut cutlets into small strips (wing-size). Heat olive oil in frying pan. Liberally dust both sides of all chicken pieces. Pan fry in oil until done. Serve with celery sticks and dressing. Makes 1 serving.

NOTE: This is a great recipe to make and bring to a cocktail party or gathering.

AVOCADO CHEESE STACK

1 slice sprouted bread
½ peeled avocado
1 oz. almond or soy cheddar cheese
Sweet clover sprouts
Creamy cucumber dressing (see recipe)

Preparations:

Spread avocado on top of toasted sprouted bread. Top with remaining ingredients. Makes 1 serving.

NOTE: You can make this a sandwich by adding another slice of bread; however this will add 14 more grams of carbs.

TUNA MELT

1 slice sprouted grain bread, toasted
4 oz. canned low-sodium tuna
2 teaspoons light-canola mayonnaise (by Spectrem Naturals)
Dash of minced onion or 1 teaspoon raw onion
Dash of celery flakes
¼ cup veggie shreds cheese (cheddar) almond, or rice cheese

Preparations:

Mix tuna with mayo, onion, and celery flakes. Place on top of toast and top with cheese. Place under broiler until cheese melts. Makes 1 serving.

NOTE: Can also be made with sardines or canned salmon, however, watch sodium content. You can always rinse fish in colander to lower sodium.

TOMATO-CABBAGE SOUP

1-28 oz. can tomato puree
6 cups water
1 small onion sliced
1-12 package frozen green beans (thawed)
½ head nappa cabbage
1 shredded carrot
1 large clove elephant garlic
1 tablespoon olive oil
½ cup water

Preparations:

In large saucepan sauté onion, carrot, cabbage, and garlic in olive oil and water until tender. Add tomatoes, water, and green beans. Bring to a low boil and simmer 30 minutes.

Makes 4-6 servings.

EGG SALAD SUPREME

2 hard boiled eggs
1 recipe Honey Mustard (minus the honey) dressing
1 celery stalk (diced)
clover sprouts
1 slice sprouted grain bread

Preparations:

Chop eggs and add celery. Add dressing and mix. Place egg salad on slice of toasted bread and top with sprouts. Makes 1 serving.

DESSERTS AND SMOOHTIE RECIPES

PEACHES AND PROTEIN SMOOTHIE

1 cup of organic peaches (frozen or fresh)
(if frozen, no ice, if fresh, 4-6 ice cubes)
½ cup water
3 Tablespoons unsweetened soy milk
2 scoops of protein powder to = 120 calories
½ to 1 packet of Stevia
dash of cinnamon (optional)

Preparations:

Place ingredients in blender and blend until creamy. Makes 1 serving.

Note: Can sub in blueberries, strawberries or cherries.

CHOCOLATE BLUEBERRY SHAKE

1 cup chocolate unsweetened soy milk
½ cup blueberries (frozen)
½ small banana
1 packet of Stevia
water, if needed

Preparations:

Combine ingredients in blender and blend until desired consistency. If too thick add water and continue blending until you reach desired consistency.

Makes 1 serving.

NOTE: This recipe is also delicious with other berries such as, strawberries or raspberries.

CHOCOLATE CHERRIES JUBILEE SHAKE

1 cup unsweetened chocolate soy milk
1 cup frozen dark cherries
1 tablespoon Hersey's unsweetened cocoa
1 packet Stevia
Water

Preparations:

Add all ingredients, except water, in blender and blend. Add water until you reach desired consistency. Makes 1 serving.

APPLE RICE-PUDDING

1½ cups water
1 spray of olive/canola oil
½ cup Basmati brown rice (not instant)
1 medium apple (peeled and chopped)
¼ cup unsweetened soy milk

½ teaspoon cinnamon
3 packets Stevia

Preparations:

Heat water and spray to a boil; add rice, apple and a dash of cinnamon. Cook covered until rice and apple absorb all water. Remove from heat and stir in soy milk, Stevia, and cinnamon. Serve warm. Can top with a drizzle of soy milk if desired. Makes 2 servings.

FAVORITE FRUIT SPICE BLEND

½ teaspoon of the following spices:
Cinnamon, nutmeg, cardamom,
Stevia

Preparations:

Combine all ingredient. Store in an air tight jar. Shake well before using.

STEWED APPLES

2 organic apples (cored and sliced with peel)
¼ teaspoon cinnamon
½ cup water

Preparations:

Place sliced apples in water with cinnamon into a 1 quart saucepan. Cover and simmer until tender. Makes 2 servings.

RAINBOWFRUITSALAD

1 cup each of the following fruits
Blueberries, strawberries,
Sliced peaches, banana, kiwi
2 tablespoon lemon juice
¼ cup all fruit preserves (any flavor)
1 packet Stevia plus

Preparations:

Place fruit preserves in a microwave safe bowl and heat until melted. Add lemon juice and Stevia; stir until well blended. Add fruit and gently toss until fruit. Serve chilled. Makes 5 servings.

BAKED PEARS WITH RASPBERRY SAUCE

2 large pears (peeled with bottoms cut off level)
2 Tablespoons all-fruit raspberry preserves (melted)
Favorite fruit spice blend
Canola oil spray
Water

Preparations:

Place pears in a glass pie dish, sprayed with canola oil spray; spray pears as well. Sprinkle spice blend on tops of pears. Pour water into baking dish until ¼ inch deep. Bake at 375 degrees, spooning liquid over pears several times during baking. Bake 35-40 minutes or until tender. Melt 2 tablespoons of raspberry preserves in a microwave safe dish; spoon over tops of pears. Serve warm. Makes 2 servings.

NOTE: Can use apples sprinkled with spices and omit the raspberry sauce for baked apples.

HARVEST APPLE DELIGHT

4 large apples (sliced to equal approx. 4 cups)
¾ cup spelt or rice flour
¾ cup old fashioned oats
2 tablespoons canola oil
1 ½ teaspoons favorite spice blend
Cooking spray

Preparations:

Spray glass 8 x 8 pan with cooking spray. Arrange sliced apples in the bottom. Mix remaining ingredients and sprinkle over apples. Bake for 30-35 minutes (or until topping browns) at 375 degrees. Makes 6 servings.

NOTE: Can sub in sliced peaches or fresh blueberries for apples.

BEVERAGES

CHERRY LEMONADE

Juice of 1 lemon
4 tablespoons concentrated black cherry juice
16 ounces water
ice cubes
1 packet Stevia/Splenda

Place all ingredients except ice, in a shaker glass and shake well until blended. Add ice and shake again. Pour into 2 glasses and garnish with lemon wedges. Makes 2 servings.

NOTE: For lemonade that's more tart you can use unsweetened cranberry juice instead of cherry.

CRANBERRY COOLER

16 ounces water or sparkling water
4 teaspoons unsweetened cranberry juice concentrate
1 packet Stevia/Splenda
Wedge of lemon or lime
Ice cubes

Preparations:

Mix all ingredients in tall glass. Serve over ice. Garnish with lemon or lime.

CHOCOLATE SOY MILK

8 ounces unsweetened soy milk
2 tablespoons of unsweetened cocoa
1 packet Stevia/Splenda

Preparations:

For best results; mix all ingredients in a blender until thoroughly mixed. Makes 1 serving.

NOTE: You can add 4-6 ice cubes to make a chocolate shake.

KEYLIME COCKTAIL

8 ounces water
¼ cup key lime juice
4 ounces club soda or sparkling water
Ice cubes
Lime wedge

Preparations:

Mix all ingredients and pour over ice. Garnish with lime wedge. Makes 1 serving.

COFFEE COOLER

8 ounces decaf coffee (prepared)
¼ cup soy creamer
1/8 teaspoon cinnamon
1 packet Stevia/Splenda
4-6 cubes

Preparations:

Add all ingredients in a blender and blend until well blended.
Makes 1 serving.

HOT CHOCOLATE SOY MILK

8 ounces unsweetened soy milk
2 tablespoons unsweetened cocoa
½ vanilla
1 packet Stevia/Splenda

Preparations:

Warm all ingredients in a small saucepan. For best results you should use a double boiler. Makes 1 serving.

NOTE: For a creamier beverage use ¼ cup soy creamer and ¾ cup of unsweetened chocolate soy milk.

GLOSSARY FOR COOKING TERMINOLOGY

Bake: To cook food uncovered in any type of oven, however, when referred to any kinds of meat, fish, or poultry, it is called roasting.

Baste: To keep food moistened during the cooking process. Melted fat drippings, juices, or sauces are the usual liquids used.

Beat: To make a mixture smooth and well blended using an electric mixer, blender, or by hand with a whisk.

Blend: To mix together, thoroughly, two or more ingredients using a blender, mixer, or by hand with a spoon.

Braises: To cook food over a low heat in a small amount of water, broth, or juice, in a covered pan.

Chop: To cut food into small pieces using a knife, chopper, blender, or food processor.

Coat: To cover food, on all sides, with flour, bread crumbs, and egg mixture, sauces, or marinades.

Dice: To cut food into tiny pieces.

Dress: To coat food (like salad) with sauces or prepared dressings, usually by tossing the food together.

Fry: To cook food over high heat in a small amount of fat.

Grill: To cook food over a bed-of-hot coals, or on an electric or gas grill. To cook over direct heat.

Pan-fry: To cook food over a high heat in a small amount of fat.

Parfait: A desert made of layers of fruit and another food, such as yogurt, jello, or pudding.

Peel: To remove outer covering of fruits or vegetables with a vegetable peeler or knife.

Poach: To cook foods over low heat in liquid.

Preheat: To heat oven, prior to baking, to the desired temperature.

Shred: To cut food into small thin pieces by using a shredded, grater, or vegetable peeled. Some food processors can also accomplish this task.

Simmer: To cook food over low-heat in a liquid that's not quite boiling.

Steam: To cook food on a rack or in a steamer basket that resembles a small colander, in a covered pan with steaming hot water.

Stir-fry: To quick-fry sliced or chopped food in either a wok or a skillet with a small amount of fat.

Toss: To lift foods gently using utensils until food is all mixed together or coated thoroughly.

Whip: To beat rapidly with a mixer or blender, or by hand with a whisk, while working in air to increase volume.

Chapter Eight

Maintaining Health, For Life

Congratulations on completing the FED program. This chapter will assist you with any questions you may have about the program's individual segments, as well as those pertaining to maintenance. I will also give you tips on how to maintain your new-found weight and health, for life.

We can incorporate many things into our lives that will further enhance our health. I encourage you to continue with the program as your primary basis for eating. You can always fall back to the first segment, if at any time you find your weight creeping back up. I encourage you to continue to use the knowledge learned during these past eight weeks. You have learned about the many obvious and hidden dangers surrounding the foods you eat. By now you know what foods will nourish the body and promote health, as well as those that will lead to disease susceptibility. This doesn't mean we can never consume those sinful foods, especially those that only satisfy our emotions and do nothing to nourish the body. It simply means that we have to utilize good judgment where these foods are concerned. Special occasions like holidays, anniversaries, and birthdays are usually our greatest challenges. We will not gain all our weight back, or suddenly come down with a chronic disorder from consuming a piece of cake with a cup of coffee, or soda. Life is to be enjoyed and eating well is not meant to be stressful. Learn to balance the two and you'll do just fine.

Balance and You

I have to say that trying to balance our lives is easier said than done. In this crazy era of hectic schedules and never having enough of time in the day, we find ourselves with more on our plate than we can handle; and I don't mean food. Many of us work two jobs or are stay-at-home moms, with to do lists a mile long. It seems we can't ever find the time to accomplish the things we have to for others; let alone for ourselves. A dear friend of mine who is a life educator, Pam Samuels, teaches a wonderful class on prioritizing. She teaches a valuable lesson on how to decipher what's important in life and what's not. If you spend all your life "doing for others," you will find that your life may just pass you by. You will miss out on so many wonderful things and all you will have are regrets for the things you didn't do or weren't able to do because you were too busy doing for others. If you were not around for those people who count on you most, they would either fend for themselves or find another care giver. In other words, without you they will go on; and life will go on. This lesson teaches us that life is too short for the constantly doing for others occupation. There are no health benefits offered for this position because the risks are too high.

By taking care of everything, but what matters the most, which is YOU, you set yourself up for all kinds of health problems. Did you know that most breast cancer patients are former caregivers and usually to a fault? I co-facilitate a breast cancer educational-support group called, A Woman's Circle of Hope and in this group are several very courageous, special ladies. To hear these ladies tell their stories about how they ran themselves into the ground, (prior to their diagnosis), either by selling their souls to their jobs, families, or parents, it all came down to their roles as care givers. Their greatest lesson was to discover who mattered most in their lives. Ideally, we should be able to learn this valuable lesson before we get sick, but unfortunately we neglect to heed the warnings.

The first priority has to be YOU. One of the analogies that Pam uses sums this up perfectly. When you are on a flight, the airline stewardess has a set list of instructions pertaining to safety. When she gets to the part that instructs those passengers that are flying with young children, you are instructed to place the oxygen mask over your face first before your secure your child's. This is to ensure that you will be better able to take care of that child if you take care of yourself first. You are, and should always be, priority number one.

Balance and Family

Now that you have realized that YOU are what matters most in YOUR life, you need to learn how to balance the rest of your life. Let's begin with family. Family is probably one of the toughest balancing acts to juggle in ones' life. We never seem to have enough time for those we love most. We are so busy trying to prove our self-worth to everyone else that we neglect those that matter most. I happen to be one of these people. I despise being told I have issues, that is, until I realize I really do have issues. We all do. Issues are an intricate part of life; also called life lessons. We don't always care to admit to them, but when we do, it's powerful; and that is the first step toward self-growth. I have been working hard at learning to say the word, 'NO' when people ask favors of me when I already have a full agenda. In the past, if I were to say yes to everyone, I would find a way to squeeze one more thing into my already busy schedule. Instead, by now learning to say no, I try to find the time for family members or matters that absolutely need my attention, such as important things like being there to talk to your spouse, children, or parents when they need advice, guidance, or just a hand to hold or a shoulder to cry on.

I can remember having a discussion with my husband, Michael, who is one of my greatest teachers, after he had one of his usual Wednesday or Sunday telephone chats with his mother Rita. I asked him why he found it necessary to stay on the phone listening to small talk for over an hour twice a week. It actually bothered me that he didn't tell her he had things to do, and that he'd catch up with her another time. Instead, he would stop whatever he was doing to take her phone calls. He simply looked at me and said, "Honey, one day those phone calls are going to stop coming in, and I won't have the chance to speak to my mother again."

Wow, talk about the proverbial slap in the face. I never in my life, felt as shallow as I did at that moment. I still cry when I remember that conversation. Rita is gone now almost two years and I can't tell you how much I miss hearing her voice. I would pay dearly for one of those silly, yet so meaningful, phone conversations. Michael always finds the time to balance family life with his own life. As for me, I am still learning this valuable lesson. If we truly are too busy to lend a helping hand, then we can't allow ourselves to feel guilty, nor can we allow others to make us feel guilty. However, if we can make the time to help out a family member or friend in need, keep in mind how much better we feel once we can accomplish that task. Doing for others can certainly have its just rewards.

Balance and the Workplace

For many of us, the workplace holds some of our greatest challenges. It is where we spend the majority of our day. I have personally found that the workplace has changed over the past few years, for the better. I have taken the FED program out into businesses to offer employees what I call an 'At Work' option. This is where I go to the place of business during the lunch hour and teach the FED program to those that are interested. I must admit that I was pleasantly surprised at the working conditions of some of these companies. One company boasted a full-working gym that was larger than my entire house, and came complete with trainers. Another company had a beautiful walking track that circled a beautiful lake with a park-like setting. Many of these businesses are incorporating wellness programs for their employees with wonderful incentive programs. I was really impressed. If you think about it, these companies are yards ahead of other businesses for a number of reasons. The main reason is that by showing an interest in the health of their employees, they are going to get more from each employee in the way of performance and attendance. They will also ideally save money when it comes to healthcare. Educating employees by means of health fairs or by implementing health programs in the workplace is a smart business strategy for both the employer and the employee.

No matter how pleasant the workplace may be, it is still the number one "stressor" in our lives. Deadlines, promotions, layoffs, new employees, new bosses, lost accounts, presentations, and missed quotas can all be very stressful situations. Stress is one of the biggest FED program challenges that we must face, and unfortunately when they occur in the workplace, there is always an accommodating vending machine around to console us. Stress is considered a primary cause of disease, often resulting because of the continuous demands that are constantly placed upon us by family, friends or work. Stress, according to the *Taber's Cyclopedic Medical Dictionary*, means any physical, physiological, or psychological force that disturbs equilibrium. As you can see, stress covers an expansive area. It can be something as simple as not being able to find your other black sock or something as devastating as the passing of a loved one. Regardless of the cause stress affects us all differently. There are some people who stop eating when they are stressed. I, on the other hand, will go right to the pantry.

We need to learn how to handle stress so that we can avoid these kinds of pitfalls. I have read many books and found that the works of great life-changing authors, like Caroline Myss, Ph.D., and Don Miguel Ruiz, helped me put life into perspective. I will include the titles of these books in my recommended reading section. I mentioned earlier how we have to learn to shut out the trivial small stuff, that doesn't seem to matter in the grand scheme of life. Instead we must concentrate on those things that matters most to us. The same principle applies when dealing with stress. If it's the small inconsequential stuff then let it go and move on. I've seen too many sick people that stayed with jobs that put them in the diseased state they're in now. Learning how to handle stress is vital to balance within the workplace.

Eating a healthy, caffeine-free diet, getting plenty of exercise, breath work, meditation, and open lines of communication are all key components of stress reduction. The FED program can help you with the first requirement. The second key component, exercise, is also a part of the program; however you can incorporate your exercise routine at work. Get out and walk to reduce stress. Fresh air and sunshine always helps stress levels, even when things seem pretty bleak. Exercise helps by allowing the busy, problem solving, over-worked half of the brain to take a backseat, giving the creative, spontaneous half of the brain the chance to take over and direct you for awhile. Many athletes can attest to the fact that during exercise is when their most creative inspirational thoughts come forth.

Breath work and meditation are two things that are easily incorporated into your work schedule. It has been proven that deep breathing can help lower blood pressure and reduce stress levels. Close your eyes and breathe in slowly to the count of seven, then slowly exhale to the count of seven. Do this exercise seven times for instant relaxation. Meditation is something we should all practice. The best time to meditate is anytime when you can quiet the mind for a few moments. For a lot of us our minds go twenty-four seven. We are the one's that need to learn the art of meditation the most. I have had the opportunity to partake in a few guided meditations and they were great and very relaxing. I would suggest that you purchase a good meditation tape or CD and listen to it until you can learn to meditate on your own. I meditate in the evening before bed and I have found that it helps me to shut down my brain, so that I can have a good nights rest. The final component to the reduction of stress is open lines of communication. This brings me to a wonderful book called, *The Four Agreements*, by Don Miguel Ruiz. One of the four agreements is, "don't make assumptions." If we don't allow ourselves to make assumptions, we will save ourselves from a whole slue of stress-related problems. Some examples follow:

Don't assume that your co-workers are going to know that you're having a bad day. Instead let co-workers know that you're in a bad mood or just having a bad day, so they won't take it personally.

Don't assume that your boss will know what you are thinking. Tell him exactly what your ideas are by expressing yourself thoroughly.

Don't assume that you are going to get that promotion. Know all the facts and know who your competition is, so you can be better prepared for the decision.

Don't assume that you have job security. Keep yourself informed and make it your business to know what's going on within and outside the company you work for.

I would suggest that you also purchase *The Four Agreements*, to find out what the other three agreements are. These too will change the way you view life. Learning to reduce the stress in your life is one of the best things you can do for disease prevention.

Balance and Life

We already discussed the importance of you; balance within the family, and in the workplace. The FED program has taught you how to eat for health and longevity, as well as taught you the importance of exercise for the body and mind. All of these crucial tools work synergistically for you to maintain balance within your life. Disease prevention is a lot more than just the food you eat or the supplements you take. You need to implement all of these aspects into your life if you want to remain disease free to live a long healthy life. Answers to questions pertaining to the FED Program and Maintenance are addressed in the next section on "Information Please." Once again, congratulations on taking control of your health by implementing the FED program into your life. Eat well, live well, and be well.

Information Please

Questions and Answers

#1

Q. I am on the first week of the program and I am experiencing a dull headache am I doing something wrong?

A. Absolutely not! This headache indicates that you are doing everything correct. This side effect is a part of the detoxification process that your body is undergoing, especially from caffeine withdrawal. It will pass in a day or two. Some people will experience fatigue as well. Make sure you are drinking all the required water to help the body flush out the many toxins you are detoxing from.

#2

Q. Do I have to drink the unsweetened cranberry juice throughout the day or can I drink the bulk of it later in the day? I am not permitted to have food or beverages in my department at work.

A. Drinking the unsweetened cranberry juice later in the day is just fine. I would prefer you to drink a little on the way to work, some during the lunch hour and while on break, and the rest while on your way home. This will save wear and tear on you kidneys, as it is better to disperse it throughout the day rather than to have to process it all at once.

#3

Q. I work two jobs and have a time management problem. I know I am doing more frozen fruits and vegetables then I should. Is this going to impede my weight loss or disease prevention progress?

A. The more fresh fruits and vegetables you can work into the program the better off you will be. I prefer fresh produce because you can wash them and the nutrient value is greater, whereas frozen vegetables have already been prepared and we have no clue how well they were washed and whether the pesticides were neutralized or not. So in answer to your question, prepare ahead and try to incorporate more fresh foods into your program. Fruits and vegetables are our disease fighters and are very important to the FED program.

#4

Q. Can I use an olive oil spray?

A. By all means. This will give you a little more versatility when it comes to cooking. Sautéing, braising, or poaching would get pretty boring if we couldn't pan fry as well. Don't overuse these sprays and I prefer you use brands that only contain the oil, soy lecithin, and a propellant. Make sure the label states that there are no chlorofluorocarbons in the product. Spectrum Naturals makes a great non-stick spray.

#5

Q. I am taking medication for high blood pressure, is there anything I should avoid as far as supplements, herbs, or food?

A. Depending on the drugs you are taking, there may be food, supplement, or herbal contraindications, as well as, drug-to-drug interactions. Your best bet is to check with an authority on these issues, like your pharmacist. In my experience grapefruit or grapefruit juice is about the only food that can interfere with hypertensive medications, however there are a several herbs to avoid if you are on hypertensive medications, like Don quai, licorice, mate, ephedra, coltsfoot, dan shen, bitter orange, hawthorn, ginsing, coleus, and epimedium.

#6

Q. I have noticed that my blood pressure has come down significantly since I started the FED program. Can I come off of my medication?

A. You will have to take this matter up with your healthcare professional; however, as far as I am concerned, you bet you can come off of your hypertensive medication. Many of my clients have already come off their blood pressure and cholesterol-lowering medications. 'Let food be your medicine, and medicine be your food' was Hippocrates' (the father of medicine) motto. I hope it will ring true for all, once again in the very near future.

#7

Q. I can't stand the taste of flaxseed oil. Is it important that I use it?

A. I would rather you stay with the flaxseed oil however, you can use flaxseed oil capsules, to be taken as a supplement if you wish. You would have to take 3 capsules 3 times daily, to equal one tablespoons of the oil. You can disguise the taste by putting it in your salad dressing (as the recipe calls for) or by putting it in your smoothie if you choose to use the oil.

#8

Q. You allow us to use spices to flavor our food in the place of salt. Can we use spice blends like a Cajun seasoning?

A. Yes, you may, however you must look at the ingredients first to make sure there is no added sugar or salt. Some of these spices are great and taste terrific but are loaded with sodium. One of my favorites is called 'Old Bay'. It contains cinnamon, red pepper, bay leaves, mustard, cloves, allspice, ginger, mace, cardamom and celery salt. Because of this last ingredient Old Bay contains sodium so use sparingly. I will recommend that you avoid it during the first two weeks of the program and then add it back in on occasion, as long as you don't overuse it. I have also purchased a product called 'salt-free Cajun seasoning' by Frontier. It has paprika, dried yeast, dehydrated onion, garlic, fennel, marjoram, thyme, cumin, and red pepper in it. It is delicious on fish or chicken. I have also added a few spice blend recipes back in chapter seven for you to try.

#9

Q. I am on ERT and Wellbutrin. I know they make me retain water; and I have gained over twenty-five pounds. My doctor now wants me to go on a diuretic but I am leery about being on so many medications. Are these medications going to keep me from losing weight?

A. This is a tough question for me because of my views concerning medications. There are several classes of drugs that cause weight gain and water retention. They are antiestrogens, antidepressants, antihistamines, hypertensives, diabetic medications, non-steroidal anti-inflammatory drugs, and tranquillizers. You are already taking two of the biggest offenders. In answer to your question, no they won't completely keep you from losing weight, however it will certainly hinder weight loss. I have several clients that have been successful at weight loss even with medications. As I mentioned in a previous chapter, my goal is to get you to where your body can once again function as it should and to eventually wean you off the medications that you will no longer need, however this is something you will have to take up with your doctor. I monitor my client's blood pressure and cholesterol throughout the program so I can see first hand how quickly blood pressure and cholesterol levels begin to drop. I would also like to mention again the contraindication between taking diuretic medications and the unsweetened cranberry juice. I have had a few clients that are taking diuretics for water retention.

After a couple of days on the FED program their ankles started swelling. I immediately took them off the cranberry juice instructing them to drink only water with lemon or lime. Cranberry is also a diuretic and is a contraindication to diuretic medications. I believe they counteract each other. Once again I will stress the importance of knowing what interactions or contraindications can occur from the medication you are taking. Unfortunately, none of my references mentioned a problem with unsweetened cranberry juice other then in relation to kidney stones. I think you are wise to be leery of medications and my advice to you is to research natural hormone replacement therapy (NHRT). A wonderful book to educate yourself on NHRT, is by Dr. John Lee and is called, "What Your Doctor May Not Have Told You About Menopause".

#10

Q. Will I ever be able to have pizza again?

A. Yes, in moderation once you have completed the program you will have learned how to incorporate foods like pizza back into your diet, as a treat –NOT as a regular staple in your diet. One large slice of pizza for example, would be your total added complex carbs, as well as your added dairy, for the day. It's all about balance.

#11

Q. Should I take a calcium supplement in addition to the calcium in the multi?

A. I do recommend additional calcium for certain people. The multi should contain about 500 mg. of supplemental calcium and the FED program (providing you consume all the food you're supposed to) averages about the same and maybe even a little more calcium. This will give you approximately 1,000-1200 mg. calcium daily. Foods like soy milk (1 cup) contains about 30 percent of your RDA, 1 oz. of almonds contains about 10 percent , ½ cup of broccoli has about 40 grams of calcium and bok choy contains as much calcium as ½ cup of milk. Other sources are sardines, other dark green leafy vegetables, eggs, salmon, walnuts, sunflower seeds, and beans. If you are a woman over fifty, or are taking medication, then I highly recommend additional calcium. Acid blockers are a big offender for blocking calcium absorption, as well as certain antibiotics, corticosteroids, diuretics, hypertensive medications, oral contraceptives and the list goes on. Women that have been taking pharmaceutical drugs chronically for years, have a high risk for osteoporosis. My mother is one of these women. Her height has decreased by almost three inches. Once again I must stress that you ask your doctor these questions, "What are the drug contraindications for this medicine and what will it do to my body?"

#12

Q. Can I use lime or orange juice in place of lemon for my alkalizing beverage?

A. You can definitely use lime juice and one of my favorites is key lime juice. Orange juice is not permitted during the first few weeks on the program. You can have orange juice in fourth week of the program, however, I will ask that you stay with either lemon or lime juice for your 'neutralizing' beverage.

#13

Q. My girlfriends and I go out dancing once a week. Should I count this as part of my exercise?

A. By all means. Any kind of physical activity counts toward the exercise requirement. Other forms of physical activities include: gardening (yard work), swimming, biking, hiking, and heavy cleaning, or perhaps joining a gym or health club. As I previously mentioned, I joined a women's exercise club called, 'Curves' and I love it. There are always other women there that are trying to lose weight or just get into better shape. We laugh, talk, and dance to the music that is constantly playing, while exercising on the equipment. It's an atmosphere that's filled with great heartfelt camaraderie. Curves, is more like a social club instead of an exercise club. They have fun contests for all to partake in and celebrate all holidays with fun activities. I highly recommend checking them out if they are in your area. Did I mention they are very reasonable?

#14

Q. I do not tolerate soy. Can I substitute in another milk product?

A. You are not alone as far as your intolerance to soy. I also have to watch how much soy I consume. Soy is not a requirement on this program, so you can sub in another milk substitute beverage. If you absolutely need a milk substitute you can use almond milk, or rice milk. Use caution with these products because of the added sugar, use sparingly. NO dairy is allowed, so milk products are out. The only time you use soy milk is in the smoothie or in decaf coffee, and it is also the milk beverage of choice in most of my recipes. I would recommend that you use the hemp protein powder if you are not going to use soy. This is to ensure that you keep to the required protein allowances. The hemp powder is made by Nutiva, and is high in protein and fiber. By making the smoothie with 2 scoops of hemp, 1 cup water, 1 cup fruit, ice cubes and Stevia, to taste, you gain the health benefits of most 'green foods' in addition to the protein and over 18 grams of fiber. This is the preferred smoothie for FED.

#15

Q. I have read that peanuts contain a toxic mold is this true? If it is true then which nuts do you recommend?

A. Peanuts are the biggest offender for molds called aflatoxins, which are carcinogenic. Peanuts are actually a legume or pea, not a nut. It is because of this mold that I do not recommend peanuts for the FED program. As far as most nuts go, buying fresh, raw, and unsalted nuts are best. Roasted nuts are altered by the roasting process, which affects the oils and the B vitamin and mineral content. Nuts should be kept in closed airtight containers and kept in the refrigerator or freezer. If left out for long periods of time they can become rancid just like certain oils. The healthiest nuts for the FED program are almonds and walnuts.

#16

Q. I am not real fond of eggs. I've had an aversion to eggs since I was a child. Is there something else I can eat instead?

A. Yes there is. If eggs are a problem either because of an allergic reaction, or a dislike for eggs, then you may substitute 2 oz. of lean protein; beef, chicken, turkey or fish + 1 teaspoon of flaxseed oil (this is in addition to the 2 tablespoons of flaxseed oil on the program). This is to replace the eggs, while still keeping with the nutrient requirements. I have found that many people don't like the yolk of the egg. Egg white omelet's are delicious and still contain over ½ the protein in the egg. So, if this is an option for you, then I suggest you give it a try. For the egg snack portion of the program, you may have 12 almonds or walnut halves.

#17

Q. If I am still hungry in the evenings, which is when my snacking habits are the worst, can I have some extra vegetables or fruit?

A. Yes, you can have all the veggies you want. Cut up raw veggies make a delicious snack. At night when I get an attack of the munchies I'll even steam up some vegetables and munch on those to satisfy my hunger. I try to save my carrot for an evening snack, because they are sweeter than most other veggies. I like to steam them and then let them cool, then spray just a little olive oil spray on them; sprinkle a little of the fruit spice blend (in the recipe section) on top and then enjoy. It makes for a nice sweet treat. Fruit I'm afraid is not an option. Only three servings of fruit daily and this includes your one serving for the smoothie.

#18

Q. I am definitely a meat eater. I have heard that buffalo is one of the highest sources of animal protein and low in fat. If this is true are we allowed to have it on the program?

A. What you heard is true. Buffalo is one of the highest sources of protein and is also very low in fat. Buffalo can be included in the program if you are adventurous and are a red meat eater. There is a mail order company called, The Perfect 10 Buffalo Ranch. You can visit them online at www.thebuffalomarket.com or call them at (402) 273-4574, they specialize in grass-fed bison.

#19

Q. Can I stay on the first segment for a few weeks if I want to lose more weight before incorporating in other foods?

A. By all means, you can take this program at your own pace and when you're ready, you can move to the next segment. Some of my clients have found that if they stay with weeks one and two for a while they will continue to lose weight. As soon as they begin to incorporate either wheat or dairy back into the diet they experience a plateau (set point). When they fall back to the first two weeks they begin losing weight again.

NOTE: You must read everything in each given program. You have to remember to increase your exercise in week four as the program states. This is very important. You have to compensate for the added calories. Some people also find that it is better to stay regimented, as in weeks one and two, in order to continue losing weight. In other words, when you start having almonds, added high glycemic fruits and complex carbs, you may find yourself getting a little lax. For example: let's say you decide to have almonds for a snack. You go to the refrigerator and take out the nuts. As you are counting out the serving of 12 nuts you unconsciously pop a few in your mouth. This serving of 12 nuts has now grown to 20. You have to stay disciplined. If any given food is too much of a temptation then don't buy it, plain and simple. As the weight starts dropping we get a false sense of security and that's when we'll get into weight gain trouble. Once you lose the desired weight and reach your goal weight, then you can reintroduce healthy favorite foods. Maintenance gives you more freedom, within reason. This program was designed to teach you how to eat without gaining weight and to educate you on unhealthy food choices that promote weight gain and disease. The FED program isn't only about losing weight; it's about achieving and maintaining good health.

#20

Q. Once I'm on the maintenance program can I have other carbs like whole grain pasta?

A. Yes, you can have pasta for an occasional treat. Very few people can have pasta without gaining weight. There is delicious ravioli that I recommend that is a lower carb choice. It's called, Pasta Fresca by TRC brands. It comes in three flavors, sun dried tomato, portabello in a spinach shell, and spinach feta cheese ravioli. They are all delicious. Total carbs are only 27 grams for 8 ravioli, fat grams are 7, and protein is 10 grams. The sodium isn't too high either, at 290 mg. per serving. I don't recommend eating pasta more than once a week.

#21

Q. Can I exercise more once I begin maintenance?

A. You should definitely exercise more on maintenance if you are consuming more calories. My rule of thumb is: if you keep your caloric intake right around your basal metabolic rate (BMR), then you should exercise no more than three times per week, however, if you increase your caloric intake by adding 200 calories daily then you can exercise up to five times weekly and still maintain your weight. It's entirely up to you. Remember, balance is the key.

#22

Q. I have been told that there are certain foods that you shouldn't eat at the same time. Can you explain why and what foods they are?

A. Certainly, these rules are called food combining. You should NOT mix protein sources at meals like steak and fish; the only exception would be eggs. Steak and eggs would be fine. The reason for this is because mixing certain proteins will hinder digestion and some combinations can actually make you very sick, becoming toxic in the body. Do NOT have carbs like bread, rice, pasta, or other grains at the same meal as proteins (meats), however, you can have a starchy vegetable with meat like corn, peas, yam, or a sweet potato. The typical American lunch is the almighty sub or sandwich, and is the worst thing for us to eat as far as digestion goes. Sandwiches break all food combining rules. No grains with meat (bread with luncheon meat), and no dairy with meat (cheese with luncheon meat). Dairy and meats should never be combined except for butter or sour cream because they are considered fats. Always eat fruit at the end of the meal or by itself, and never eat fruit with vegetables. That about covers the food combining rules.

#23

Q. What do you recommend to eat when dining out, as far as the healthiest safest foods?

A. Ah, this is a tough one, as far as some restaurants go. I stick to steak houses like Outback or Longhorn, because they usually have something I can eat on the menu. I personally order either the fresh catch of the day, or the salmon, which is usually a staple item in these types of places. I know free-range meats aren't an option in most restaurants, so I stay away from chicken and I don't consume beef. I order my fish either grilled or blackened and order a side salad and extra veggies (hold the butter). I always bring my own salad dressing, and I ask them to hold the bread please. Chinese food is pretty easy if you order the dieter's special, or ask them to hold the sauce because that's where the hidden sodium and fat is. Chicken with veggies or shrimp with veggies are your best bets when ordering Chinese food. Italian is difficult because of carb overload and Mexican is high in sodium and fat. And as I mentioned before a treat every now and then isn't going to bring all your weight back overnight.

#24

Q. I come from a large Italian family of food pushers. How can I go home to visit them without gaining all my weight back? I love them and don't want to offend them, but they don't seem to understand the words, "No Thank You." Can you give me some advice?

A. I must admit that this used to be a big problem for me too, whenever I went back home for a visit. I finally got to the point where I had to be firm. I explained that I chose to watch my weight, and am very selective when it comes to the foods I'll eat. I make it a point to thank them for offering but then politely decline. I also make it a point to ask if there is anything (food wise) that I can bring. I will usually bring something that I know I will eat.

#25

Q. What do I do once I complete the FED eight-week program, if I still have weight to lose?

A. Continue the program for as long as you need to, until you reach your desired weight. Once you reach goal you can gradually add back in healthy choices of your favorite foods. I hope that you learned (from the FED program), which foods to avoid for health reasons. Weigh yourself regularly to monitor your weight. If at any time you see that your weight is going up, drop back to the first two weeks of the program. The same advice goes for vacations or holidays.

I hope these answers helped to tie up any lose ends for you. These are questions that were posed to me during my FED program lectures. If there is something that you don't understand about the FED program, just do 'your personal best', and you'll be fine. On the following pages you will find a resource list of companies that I have personally dealt with. Good luck and I wish you continued success with your weight loss and your journey toward disease prevention. Eat well, live well, and be well!

Glossary

Antigen – Any substance that, when introduced into the body, causes the formation of antibodies against it.

Antihypertensive – A drug or substance that lowers blood pressure.

Antioxidant – A compound that prevents free-radical, or oxidative damage.

Basal Metabolic Rate – The rate of metabolism when the body is at rest.

Beta-carotene – A plant carotene that can be converted to two vitamin A molecules.

Blood Pressure – The force exerted by the blood as it presses against blood vessels and attempts to stretch the vessels.

Bromelain – An enzyme with protein-digesting properties, that is found in pineapple.

Calorie – A unit of heat. A calorie is the amount of heat that it takes to raise 1 kg. of water to 1 degree C.

Candida Albicans – Yeast that is usually found in the intestinal tract.

Carbohydrate – One of a group of substances including sugars, starches, glycogen, dextrins, and cellulose.

Carcinogen – A cancer-causing agent.

Celiac's disease – Also called celiac sprue and gluten, sensitive enteropothy is a digestive disorder that is caused by a hereditary intolerance to gluten. The body treats gluten as if it was an antigen and launches an attack causing damage to the digestive tract.

Corticosteroids – A class of drugs primarily used to treat inflammatory conditions and to suppress the immune system.

Dehydration – Excessive loss of water from the body.

Diastolic Pressure – The measurement of the pressure in the arteries during the rest phase of the heartbeat. The bottom number - Example: 120/80, 80 is the diastolic number.

Diuretic– A compound that can be food, supplement or drug that causes increased urination.

Enzyme – An organic catalyst that changes the rate of a chemical reaction.

Essential fatty acids – Fatty acids are acids that the body cannot manufacture. Lenolenic and lenoleic acids. Also known as omega 3 and omega 6.

Estrogens – Hormones that exert female characteristics.

Free radical – Highly reactive molecules that are characterized by an unpaired electron, that can bind to and destroy, cellular compounds.

Glucose – A monosaccharide found in the blood. One of the prime energy sources for the body.

Gluten – A protein found in wheat and some other grains.

Holistic Medicine – A modality that involves treating the whole person not just their symptoms, or the body parts in which they occur.

Hormone – A secretion of an endocrine gland that controls and regulatesfunctions within the body.

Hyperglycemia – High blood sugar.

Hypoglycemia – Low blood sugar.

Hypotention – Low blood pressure.

Insulin – A hormone that is secreted by the pancreas that lowers blood sugar levels.

Lactose – One of the sugars present in milk.

Lipids – Fats, phospholipids, steroids, and prostaglandins.

Lymph – Fluid contained in lymphatic vessels that flow through the lymphatic system to be returned to the blood.

Malabsorption – The impairment of the absorption of nutrients.

Metabolism – A term for all the chemical processes that take place within the body.

Mucus – The slick, slimmy fluid secreted by the mucus membranes which act as a lubricant and protector of mucus membranes.

Neurotransmitters – Substances that modify or transmit nerve impulse transmission.

Papain – An enzyme that aids the digestion of protein found in papaya.

Pathogen – Any agent, particularly a microorganism that causes disease.

Peristalsis – Muscular contractions in succession, that takes place in the intestines, moving food through the intestinal tract.

Physiology – The study of the functioning of the body.

Phytoestrogens – Plant compounds that have estrogenic effects.

Prostaglandins – Hormone-like compounds that are manufactured from essential fatty acids.

Saturated fat – A fat found in animal products such as meat, milk, milk products, and eggs.

Trans fatty acid – The fats found in margarine. Hydrogenated oils.

Vitamin – An essential compound necessary to act as a catalyst, in normal processes of the body.

Western diet – A diet characterized of western cultures. A diet high in fat, low in fiber, high in sugar and carbohydrates, and processed foods.

Resources

This is a list of resources that I have put together for your convenience. These are companies that I have either used firsthand, or have used their products. Feel free to contact them for any information you may need.

Health Shops

Native Sun
10000 San Jose Blvd.
Jacksonville, FL. 32257
(904) 260-6950

Local Jacksonville organic grocery store. Featuring organic produce and other food items. Free-range meats are available in store and for ordering. Native Sun also features a juice bar and full deli. Supplements, herbs, books, cosmetics and pet supplies are also available.

The Health Shoppe
12620-16 Beach Blvd.
Jacksonville, FL. 32246
(904) 641-4410

Local Jacksonville health shop. Supplements, homeopathics, grocery items, and books.

The Natural Medicine Shoppe
1891 Beach Blvd.
Jacksonville Beach, FL. 32250
(904 249-4372

Local Jacksonville health shop featuring a compound pharmacy, herbs, supplements, organic grocery items, organic wines, and homeopathics.

GNC Stores
(Check your area for local stores)

Health stores nation wide. Supplements, herbs, and protein powders.

Practitioners

Stephen Grable, M.D.
Complementary Care Center
1504 Roberts Dr.
Jacksonville Beach, FL. 32250
(904) 247-7455

Complimentary medicine physician. Offering conventional and alternative health options.

Valerie Miles, M.D., P.A.
4311 Salisbury Rd.
Jacksonville, FL. 32256
(904) 338-0434

Board certified in conventional and holistic medicine. Pediatrics specialist.

Cleveland W. Randolph Jr., M.D.
1891 Beach Blvd.
Jacksonville Beach, FL. 32250
(904) 249-3743

OBGYN that specializes in Natural Hormone Replacement therapy. Compound pharmacist with a pharmacy on the premises.

Mail Order Health Foods

Sun Organic Farm
P.O. Box 2429
Valley Center, CA. 92082
(888) 269-9888
www.sunorganic.com

A great source for nuts, seeds, grains, dried fruits, snacks and more.

Walnut Acres
Penns Creek, PA. 17862
(800)433-3998

A wonderful company for ordering natural foods. Sauces, vegetables, juices and many other items available.

Eden Foods, Inc.
701 Tecumseh Road
Clinton, MI 49236
(888) 424-3336
www.edenfoods.com

Natural food products for mail ordering.

Spectrum Naturals
133 A Copeland
Petaluma, CA. 94952
(707) 778-8900

Good mail order source for olive, canola, and flaxseed oils.

Jason's Natural Cosmetics
8468 Warner Drive
Culver City, CA. 90232
(800) 527-6605

www.jason-natural.com

I have tried several products from Jason's and love them all. Moisturizing creams, lotions, soaps, shampoos and cosmetics.

Supplements & Herbs

Boiron
6 Campus Blvd. Building A
Newtown Square, PA. 19073
(800) Blu-Tube

Homeopathic remedies and supplies. A terrific homeopathic flu remedy I use whenever I travel is 'Oscillococcinum'. Boiron is the manufacturer.

Country Life
101 Corporate Drive
Hauppage, NY. 11788
(631) 231-1031
www.country-life.com

Full line of supplements, herbs, teas, oils, and, Biocem Sports and Fitness products.

Natren's
3105 Willow /lake
Westlake Village, CA. 91361
(800) 992-3323
www.natren.com

One of the best companies for probiotics.

Natrol Inc.
21411 Prairie Street
Chatsworth, CA. 91311
(800) 326-1520

www.natrol.com

Supplements. DHEA, Ester C with bioflavonoids, as well as digestive enzymes.

Nature's Way
10 Mountain Springs Pkwy.
Springville, UT. 84663
(800) 962-8873
www.naturesway.com

Herbal remedies, probiotics, and supplements.

Solaray
1400 Kearns Blvd.
Park City, UT. 84060
(800) 669-8877
www.nutraceutical.com/solaray.cfm

Great source for herbal blends.

Solgar Vitamin and Herb Company
500 Willow Tree Rd.
Leonia, NJ. 07605
(877) 765-4274

Full line of supplements.

References & Suggested Reading

1. Samuel S. Epstein, M.D., *The Politics Of Cancer, Revisited* (USA East Ridge Press, 1998).

2. Phyllis A. Balch, CNC, James T. Balch, M.D., *Prescription For Nutritional Healing* (Penguin Putnam Inc., 2000).

3. David Steinman & Samuel S. Epstein, M.D., *The Safe Shopper's Bible* (Macmillan USA,1995).

4. J. Robert Hatherhill, Ph.D., *Eat To Beat Cancer*, (Renaissance Books, 1998).

5. Elson M. Haas, M.D., *Staying Healthy With Nutrition,* Celestial Arts Publishing, 1992).

6. Ann Louise Gittleman, *The Fat Flush Plan,* (McGraw-Hill, 2002).

7. Jennie Brand-Miller, PhD., Thomas M.S. Wolever, M.D., PhD., Kay Foster-Powell, M. Nutr. & Diet, Stephen Colgiuri M.D., *The New Glucose Revolution* (Marlowe & Company, 1999).

8. Russell L. Blaylock, M.D., *Excitotoxins, The Taste That Kills,* (Health Press, 1997).

9. *Taber's Cyclopedic Medical Dictionary*, (F.A. Davis, 2001).

10. John R. Smythies, M.D., *Every Person's Guide To Antioxidants,* (John R. Smythies, 1998).

11. Stephanie Beling, M.D., *Power Foods* (Harper Collins Publisher's, 1997).

12. Michael Murray, N.D., Joseph Pizzorno, N.D. *Encyclopedia of Natural Medicine Revised 2nd Addition* (Joseph Pizzorno and Michael T. Murray, 1998).

13. Schuyler W. Lininger, Jr. DC, Alan R. Gaby, M.D., Steve Austin, N.D., Forrest Batz, Pharm D, Eric Yarnell, N.D., Donald J. Brown, N.D. and George Constantine, RPh., PhD., *A-Z Guide To Drug-Herb-Vitamin Interactions* (Healthnotes Inc., 1999).

14. Michael Snayerson, Mark Plotkin, *The Killers Within*, (Little, Brown, and Co. 2002).

15. Caroline Myss, Ph.D, Norman Shealy, M.D., *The Creation of Health,* (Crown Publishing Group, 1988, 1993).

16. Don Miguel Ruiz, *The Four Agreements*, (Amber-Allen Publishing, 1997).

Printed in the United States
99230LV00008B/182/A

9 781413 754476